METABOLISM RESET DIET FOR ENDOMORPH WOMEN

Revitalize Your Liver Health And Halt Fat Storage By Losing Weight Naturally

Christiana Vince and Davis Cruise

TABLE OF CONTENTS

INTRODUCTION

Welcome, fellow endomorph ladies, to the grand adventure of resetting your metabolism! Picture this: You're sitting there, pondering life's mysteries, maybe with a snack in hand (no judgment here!), and you stumble upon this book titled "Metabolism Reset Diet for Endomorph Women." You raise an eyebrow, intrigued yet cautiously optimistic. Could this be the magical solution you've been searching for? Well, my friend, you've come to the right place. Buckle up, because we're about to embark on a journey filled with laughter, sweat, delicious food, and yes, even a few tears (but hopefully tears of joy).

Now, before we dive headfirst into the nitty-gritty details of metabolism and meal planning, let's take a moment to acknowledge something important: being an endomorph woman ain't always a walk in the park. Trust me, I get it. We live in a world where "one-size-fits-all" diets reign supreme, and societal pressures to look a certain way can feel downright suffocating at times. It's like trying to fit a square peg into a round hole, am I right?

But fear not, my lovely endomorph comrades, because this book is not about conforming to unrealistic standards or depriving ourselves of the pleasures of life (cue dramatic music). Nope, it's about embracing our unique bodies, understanding how they work, and making choices that nourish us from the inside out. Think of it as a love letter to your metabolism, if you will—a gentle nudge in the right direction, sprinkled with a dash of tough love and a whole lot of compassion.

So, what exactly can you expect from this metabolism reset extravaganza? Well, let me break it down for you. We're going to start by getting cozy with the science behind metabolism and why it behaves the way it does in us endomorph gals. Spoiler alert: it's not because we're lazy or lack willpower (seriously, can we retire that tired old stereotype already?). Then, we'll roll up our sleeves and set some kick-ass goals for ourselves—because let's face it, nothing feels better than crushing those goals like a boss lady.

Next up, we'll take a long, hard look at our current diet and lifestyle habits. And hey, I won't judge if you've got a secret stash of chocolate hidden in the pantry (been there, done that). The important thing is that we're honest with ourselves about where we're at so we can figure out where we want to go. From there, we'll dive into the nuts and bolts of the metabolism reset diet, exploring everything from essential nutrients to meal planning tips and sample recipes that will make your taste buds sing with joy.

But wait, there's more! We're not just going to talk about food—we're also going to get our sweat on with some killer workouts designed specifically for us endomorph ladies. Because let's be real, exercise is about way more than just burning calories—it's about feeling strong, confident, and downright fabulous in our own skin.

Of course, no journey would be complete without a few bumps in the road, right? That's why we'll also tackle some of the common challenges that come with resetting your metabolism, like dealing with cravings, overcoming plateaus, and navigating those pesky emotional eating triggers. But fear not, my friends, because I've got your back every step of the way.

And hey, speaking of bumps in the road, let's not forget to celebrate the victories—big and small—along the way. Whether it's dropping a dress size, nailing that new yoga pose, or simply feeling more energized and alive than ever before, every little win deserves a round of applause (and maybe a victory dance or two).

So, my fellow endomorph warriors, are you ready to embark on this epic quest to reset your metabolism and reclaim your health and happiness? If your answer is a resounding "heck yes!" then grab your favorite snack (because hey, life's too short to eat boring food) and let's dive in. Together, we'll laugh, we'll sweat, we'll eat our veggies (and maybe a slice of cake or two), and most importantly, we'll embrace every step of this wild and wonderful journey. Let's do this!

Understanding Endomorph Body Types

Endomorphs have softer bodies with curves. They have a wide waist and hips and large bones, though they may or may not be overweight. Their weight is often in their hips, thighs, and lower abdomen. Endomorphs often have lots of body fat and muscle and tend to gain weight easily.

The endomorph body type stands out as one with its own distinctive characteristics and challenges. But what exactly defines an endomorph, and how does understanding this body type empower us on our journey to optimal health and wellness? Let's embark on a journey of self-discovery and exploration as we delve into the nuances of endomorph body types.

Unveiling the Endomorph Identity

First and foremost, let's dispel any misconceptions or stereotypes surrounding the term "endomorph." Contrary to popular belief, being an endomorph is not a condemnation to a life of perpetual struggle with weight management. Rather, it's simply a reflection of our genetic predisposition towards certain physical traits, such as a rounded figure, a tendency to store fat more readily, and a slower metabolism.

It's important to approach the concept of endomorphism with a sense of curiosity and acceptance, rather than judgment or self-criticism. After all, our bodies are magnificent vessels that carry us through life's adventures, and each body type comes with its own set of strengths and vulnerabilities. Embracing our endomorph identity is the first step towards understanding and honoring our bodies for the incredible beings they are.

The Science Behind Endomorphism

At the heart of understanding endomorph body types lies the science of genetics and metabolism. Endomorphism is believed to be influenced by a combination of genetic factors, hormonal fluctuations, and lifestyle choices. While genetics play a significant role in determining our body type, it's essential to recognize that they are not the sole determinants of our destiny.

Hormones, such as insulin and cortisol, also play a crucial role in shaping our metabolic profile and body composition. For endomorphs, the delicate balance of these hormones can sometimes tilt in favor of fat storage, leading to challenges in weight management and insulin sensitivity. Understanding the interplay between genetics and hormones empowers us to make informed choices that support our metabolic health and overall well-being.

Navigating the Challenges of Endomorphism

It's no secret that life as an endomorph comes with its fair share of challenges. From societal pressures to conform to unrealistic beauty standards to the frustration of trying to lose weight despite seemingly endless efforts, the journey can sometimes feel like an uphill battle. But here's the thing: you are not alone.

By acknowledging and embracing our endomorph identity, we can shift our perspective from one of defeat to one of empowerment. Instead of viewing our bodies as obstacles to overcome, we can choose to see them as allies on our journey towards health and vitality. This shift in mindset opens up a world of possibilities, where we can approach our health goals with compassion, curiosity, and resilience.

Harnessing the Power of Nutrition and Exercise

One of the keys to thriving as an endomorph lies in finding the right balance of nutrition and exercise that supports our unique metabolic needs. While there is no one-size-fits-all approach, there are certain strategies that endomorphs may find particularly beneficial. For example, focusing on a diet rich in whole, nutrient-dense foods can help stabilize blood sugar levels and promote satiety, reducing the risk of overeating and weight gain.

Similarly, incorporating a combination of strength training and cardiovascular exercise can help boost metabolism, build lean muscle mass, and improve insulin sensitivity. By tailoring our nutrition and exercise routines to our individual needs, we can optimize our metabolic health and achieve lasting results.

The Importance of Tailored Nutrition for Endomorph Women

When it comes to endomorph women, the importance of tailored nutrition takes on a whole new level of significance. As we embark on this journey of self-discovery and empowerment, let's delve into the intricacies of how tailored nutrition can unlock the full potential of our metabolic health.

Understanding the Endomorph Advantage

Before we dive into the specifics of tailored nutrition, let's take a moment to appreciate the unique advantages that endomorph women bring to the table. While it's true that we may have a predisposition towards storing fat more readily, we also possess an incredible capacity for strength, resilience, and vitality. Our bodies are finely tuned machines, capable of adapting to a wide range of environments and challenges.

By reframing our perception of endomorphism as a strength rather than a weakness, we can begin to harness the full potential of our metabolic prowess. Instead of viewing ourselves through the lens of societal expectations or arbitrary beauty standards, let's celebrate the incredible diversity of our bodies and the endless possibilities they hold.

The Pitfalls of One-Size-Fits-All Nutrition

In a world inundated with fad diets and quick-fix solutions, it's easy to fall into the trap of adopting a one-size-fits-all approach to nutrition. But here's the thing: what works for one person may not necessarily work for another, especially when it comes to endomorph women. Our bodies have unique metabolic needs and preferences, and a cookie-cutter approach to nutrition simply won't cut it.

When we try to force our bodies into a mold that doesn't fit, we run the risk of wreaking havoc on our metabolism, hormones, and overall well-being. Crash diets, extreme calorie restriction, and overly restrictive eating patterns may yield short-term results, but they rarely lead to sustainable, long-term success. It's time to break free from the shackles of diet culture and embrace a more nuanced, personalized approach to nutrition.

The Power of Personalized Nutrition

Enter tailored nutrition: a game-changing approach that takes into account our individual metabolic needs, preferences, and goals. Instead of blindly following the latest diet craze, tailored nutrition empowers us to become the architects of our own health destiny. It's about listening to our bodies, tuning into our hunger and satiety cues, and making choices that nourish us from the inside out.

For endomorph women, personalized nutrition may involve focusing on nutrient-dense, whole foods that support metabolic health and promote satiety. It may mean experimenting with different macronutrient ratios to find what works best for our bodies. It may even involve seeking guidance from a qualified nutrition professional who can help us navigate the complexities of our unique physiology.

The Path to Lasting Transformation

But perhaps most importantly, tailored nutrition is not just about what we eat—it's about how we nourish our bodies, minds, and souls. It's about cultivating a healthy relationship with food, free from guilt, shame, or restriction. It's about honoring our bodies as the incredible vessels they are, and fueling them with love, respect, and compassion.

UNDERSTANDING ENDOMORPH METABOLISM

Exploring the Characteristics of Endomorphs

Endomorphs tend to have a softer, rounder physique, with a tendency to store fat more readily than other body types. This is often accompanied by a wider bone structure and a higher percentage of body fat, giving endomorphs a more voluptuous appearance.

But here's the thing: our body composition is not something to be ashamed of or judged. It's simply a reflection of our genetic blueprint and the intricate dance of hormones and metabolism that governs our physiology. By embracing our unique body composition with curiosity and acceptance, we can begin to unlock the full potential of our health and well-being.

The Metabolic Puzzle of Endomorphs

When it comes to metabolism, endomorphs have a few tricks up their sleeves that set them apart from other body types. One of the key characteristics of endomorph metabolism is its tendency to be slower and more efficient at storing energy. This means that endomorphs may have a harder time burning calories and may be more prone to weight gain if not careful.

But here's the good news: our metabolism is not set in stone. With the right approach to nutrition, exercise, and lifestyle, we can optimize our metabolic health and achieve our health and fitness goals. It's all about understanding our unique metabolic profile and making choices that support our body's natural tendencies.

Embracing Strength and Resilience

Despite the challenges that come with being an endomorph, there are also many strengths and advantages to celebrate. Endomorphs are often blessed with incredible strength, resilience, and endurance, making us well-suited for activities that require power and stamina. Our bodies have an amazing capacity for adaptation and growth, allowing us to thrive in a wide range of environments and circumstances.

How Metabolism Differs in Endomorph Women

For endomorph women, the metabolism plays a unique and often misunderstood role, shaping our bodies and influencing our health in profound ways. Join me on a journey of exploration as we unravel the mysteries of how metabolism differs in endomorph women and embrace the power of our metabolic prowess.

The Metabolic Blueprint of Endomorph Women

At the heart of understanding how metabolism differs in endomorph women lies a deeper appreciation for the intricate interplay of hormones, genetics, and lifestyle factors. Endomorph women are blessed with a metabolism that is finely attuned to the art of energy storage, thanks to a combination of genetic factors and hormonal fluctuations.

Unlike our ectomorph and mesomorph counterparts, who may have faster metabolisms and an easier time burning calories, endomorph women often find themselves grappling with a slower metabolic rate and a tendency to store fat more readily. But here's the thing: our metabolism is not our destiny. With the right approach to nutrition, exercise, and lifestyle, we can optimize our metabolic health and achieve our health and fitness goals.

Hormonal Influences on Metabolism

One of the key factors that differentiate the metabolism of endomorph women is the delicate dance of hormones that govern our physiological processes. Hormones such as insulin, cortisol, and estrogen play a crucial role in regulating metabolism, appetite, and fat storage, and can have a profound impact on our metabolic health.

For endomorph women, hormonal imbalances or fluctuations may tip the scales in favor of fat storage, leading to challenges in weight management and insulin sensitivity. But by understanding the role that hormones play in our metabolism, we can begin to make informed choices that support hormonal balance and optimize our metabolic health.

The Role of Lifestyle Factors

In addition to genetics and hormones, lifestyle factors also play a significant role in shaping the metabolism of endomorph women. Factors such as diet, physical activity, stress levels, and sleep quality can all influence metabolic rate and energy balance, and can either support or hinder our metabolic health.

For endomorph women, adopting a balanced and sustainable approach to nutrition and exercise is key to optimizing metabolic health. This may involve focusing on nutrient-dense, whole foods that support stable blood sugar levels and promote satiety, as well as incorporating a combination of strength training and cardiovascular exercise to boost metabolism and build lean muscle mass.

Common Challenges Faced by Endomorphs in Weight Management

Endomorphs often find themselves in spaces filled with unique challenges and obstacles. But what are these challenges, and how do they impact our journey towards optimal health and wellness? Join me as we shine a light on the common hurdles faced by endomorphs in weight management and explore strategies for overcoming them with grace and resilience.

1. Slower Metabolism

At the top of the list of challenges for endomorphs is the reality of having a slower metabolism compared to other body types. Endomorphs often find themselves burning calories at a slower rate, making weight loss more challenging and requiring a greater degree of diligence and patience.

2. Tendency to Store Fat

Another common challenge for endomorphs is their propensity to store fat more readily than other body types. This means that even small dietary indiscretions or periods of inactivity can lead to noticeable increases in body fat, making weight management a constant balancing act.

3. Difficulty in Losing Belly Fat

Endomorphs are also more likely to carry excess weight around their midsection, often manifesting as stubborn belly fat. This type of fat, known as visceral fat, is not only unsightly but also poses serious health risks, including increased risk of heart disease, diabetes, and other metabolic disorders.

4. Hormonal Imbalances

Hormonal imbalances can also pose a significant challenge for endomorphs in weight management. Fluctuations in hormones such as insulin, cortisol, and estrogen can disrupt metabolic function, leading to weight gain and difficulty in losing weight, particularly around the midsection.

5. Cravings and Emotional Eating

Endomorphs may also struggle with cravings and emotional eating, particularly in response to stress, boredom, or negative emotions. This can lead to overeating and weight gain, further exacerbating the challenges of weight management.

Navigating the Challenges

While the challenges faced by endomorphs in weight management may seem daunting, they are by no means insurmountable. With the right approach and mindset, it is possible to overcome these obstacles and achieve lasting success in our health and wellness journey.

Strategies for Success

1. **Focus on Whole Foods:** Instead of relying on processed and refined foods, prioritize whole, nutrient-dense foods that nourish your body and support metabolic health.

2. **Balanced Nutrition:** Aim for a balanced diet that includes a mix of protein, carbohydrates, and healthy fats to keep you feeling satisfied and energized throughout the day.

3. **Regular Exercise:** Incorporate regular exercise into your routine, focusing on both cardiovascular exercise and strength training to boost metabolism and build lean muscle mass.

4. **Stress Management:** Practice stress management techniques such as meditation, yoga, or deep breathing exercises to help mitigate the impact of stress on hormonal balance and weight management.

5. **Mindful Eating:** Practice mindful eating techniques to become more attuned to your body's hunger and satiety cues, and to reduce the likelihood of emotional eating and cravings.

SETTING GOALS FOR YOUR METABOLISM RESET

Identifying Personal Health and Wellness Goals

At the heart of identifying personal health and wellness goals lies the power of intention—the conscious decision to align our actions with our deepest desires and values. It's about taking a proactive approach to our health and well-being, rather than simply reacting to external circumstances or societal pressures.

By setting clear and meaningful goals, we create a roadmap for success—a guiding light that illuminates the path ahead and empowers us to take deliberate action towards our dreams. Whether it's improving our physical fitness, nourishing our bodies with wholesome foods, or cultivating a sense of inner peace and balance, our goals serve as beacons of inspiration and motivation on our journey towards health and happiness.

Reflecting on What Matters Most

But before we can set meaningful goals, we must first take the time to reflect on what truly matters most to us. What are our deepest desires, aspirations, and values when it comes to our health and well-being? What do we hope to achieve, experience, or embody in our quest for vitality and fulfillment?

This process of self-reflection is essential for gaining clarity and insight into our personal health and wellness goals. It allows us to connect with our inner wisdom and intuition, tapping into the infinite wellspring of potential that resides within each of us. By listening to the whispers of our hearts and honoring our deepest truths, we can uncover the goals that resonate most deeply with our souls.

Setting SMART Goals

Once we've identified our personal health and wellness goals, it's time to transform them into actionable objectives that propel us forward on our journey. This is where the concept of SMART goals comes into play—goals that are Specific, Measurable, Achievable, Relevant, and Time-bound.

Specific goals provide clarity and focus, Measurable goals allow us to track our progress and celebrate our successes, Achievable goals are realistic and within our reach, Relevant goals align with our values and priorities, and Time-bound goals have a clear deadline or timeline for completion.

By applying the SMART criteria to our health and wellness goals, we transform them from lofty aspirations into concrete action plans that propel us towards success. Whether it's committing to exercising three times a week, incorporating more fruits and vegetables into our diet, or dedicating time each day for self-care and relaxation, SMART goals provide the framework for sustainable change and transformation.

Establishing Realistic Expectations for Progress

In the pursuit of our health and wellness goals, it's easy to get swept up in the excitement of possibility and potential. We envision ourselves transformed—fitter, healthier, happier than ever before. But amidst the optimism, it's important to ground ourselves in reality and establish realistic expectations for progress. Join me as we explore the art of setting achievable goals and embracing the journey of transformation with grace and patience.

The Pitfalls of Unrealistic Expectations

Before we delve into the process of establishing realistic expectations, let's first acknowledge the dangers of setting the bar too high. Unrealistic expectations can set us up for disappointment, frustration, and even burnout. When we expect too much too soon, we set ourselves up for failure, leading to feelings of inadequacy and self-doubt.

Moreover, unrealistic expectations can also lead us down the slippery slope of comparison, as we measure our progress against unrealistic standards set by others. This can erode our self-esteem and undermine our confidence, making it even harder to stay motivated and committed to our goals.

The Importance of Patience and Persistence

In contrast to unrealistic expectations, establishing realistic expectations for progress is all about embracing the journey with patience and persistence. It's about recognizing that meaningful change takes time and effort, and that progress is not always linear. There will be ups and downs, setbacks and breakthroughs, but through it all, we must remain steadfast in our commitment to our goals.

Patience is not about passively waiting for results to magically appear—it's about trusting the process and staying the course, even when the going gets tough. It's about celebrating small victories along the way, acknowledging the progress we've made, and staying focused on the bigger picture.

Setting Milestones and Celebrating Progress

One of the keys to establishing realistic expectations for progress is to set meaningful milestones along the way. These milestones serve as checkpoints on our journey, allowing us to track our progress and celebrate our achievements. Whether it's losing a certain amount of weight, hitting a new personal best in the gym, or adopting a healthier eating habit, milestones provide tangible evidence of our progress and keep us motivated and inspired.

But it's important to remember that progress is not always measured in pounds lost or inches gained. Sometimes, the most meaningful progress is internal—a shift in mindset, a newfound sense of confidence, a deeper connection to our bodies and ourselves. By broadening our definition of progress, we open ourselves up to a world of possibilities and potential.

Cultivating Self-Compassion and Resilience

Establishing realistic expectations for progress requires us to cultivate a sense of self-compassion and resilience. We must be kind to ourselves, especially in moments of struggle and setback. Instead of berating ourselves for not meeting our goals, we must offer ourselves the same kindness and understanding that we would offer to a dear friend.

Creating a Vision for Your Ideal Health and Fitness

At the core of creating a vision for our ideal health and fitness lies the power of visualization—the ability to imagine and embody the life we want to live. Visualization is more than just wishful thinking; it's a powerful tool for transformation that harnesses the creative power of our minds to manifest our dreams into reality.

By taking the time to visualize our ideal state of health and fitness, we tap into our subconscious desires and motivations, clarifying our intentions and setting the stage for meaningful change. Whether it's envisioning ourselves as strong, energetic, and resilient or picturing ourselves engaging in activities we love with ease and joy, visualization provides the foundation for creating a compelling vision.

Clarifying Your Values and Priorities

Before we can craft a vision for our ideal health and fitness, we must first clarify our values and priorities. What matters most to us when it comes to our health and well-being? Is it feeling strong and confident in our bodies? Is it having the energy to pursue our passions and dreams? Is it nurturing our mental and emotional well-being?

By reflecting on our values and priorities, we gain clarity on what truly drives us and inspires us to take action. This clarity allows us to create a vision that is authentic and aligned with our deepest desires, setting the stage for sustainable and fulfilling change.

Defining Your Goals and Objectives

Once we've clarified our values and priorities, it's time to translate them into concrete goals and objectives. What specific outcomes do we want to achieve in our journey towards ideal health and fitness? Do we want to lose weight, build strength, improve flexibility, or enhance overall well-being?

By defining clear and actionable goals, we transform our vision into a roadmap for success—a series of steps and milestones that guide us towards our desired destination. Whether it's committing to a regular exercise routine, adopting healthier eating habits, or prioritizing self-care and relaxation, our goals provide direction and purpose in our health and fitness journey.

Harnessing the Power of Affirmations and Mantras

In addition to visualization and goal-setting, affirmations and mantras can serve as powerful tools for reinforcing our vision and instilling a sense of confidence and belief in our abilities. Affirmations are positive statements that affirm our desired outcomes, while mantras are short phrases or words that we repeat to ourselves as reminders of our intentions.

For example, we might use affirmations such as "I am strong and capable of achieving my fitness goals" or mantras such as "Health and vitality are my birthright" to cultivate a positive mindset and overcome self-doubt. By integrating affirmations and mantras into our daily practice, we strengthen our resolve and stay focused on our vision.

ASSESSING YOUR CURRENT DIET AND LIFESTYLE

Food Diary: Understanding Your Eating Patterns

In the journey towards optimal health and well-being, the food we consume plays a pivotal role. But how often do we truly stop to examine our eating habits and patterns? Join me as we delve into the practice of keeping a food diary—a powerful tool for understanding our eating patterns, identifying areas for improvement, and cultivating a healthier relationship with food.

The Power of Awareness

At the heart of keeping a food diary lies the power of awareness—the ability to shine a light on our eating habits and patterns with clarity and objectivity. When we keep a food diary, we create a space for mindfulness and reflection, allowing us to become more conscious of what, when, and why we eat.

By bringing awareness to our eating habits, we gain valuable insights into our behaviors and tendencies, uncovering patterns that may be contributing to our health and well-being. Whether it's mindless snacking, emotional eating, or irregular meal times, a food diary helps us to see our eating habits with fresh eyes and empowers us to make positive changes.

Getting Started

Keeping a food diary is simple and straightforward—all you need is a notebook or a smartphone app to record your meals and snacks throughout the day. Be sure to include details such as what you ate, when you ate it, where you were, and how you were feeling at the time. The more detailed your entries, the better insight you'll gain into your eating patterns.

It's also important to be honest and non-judgmental in your food diary entries. Remember, the purpose of keeping a food diary is not to criticize or punish yourself for your eating habits, but rather to gain insight and understanding into your relationship with food. Approach your food diary with curiosity and compassion, and use it as a tool for self-discovery and growth.

Identifying Eating Patterns

As you continue to keep your food diary, you'll begin to notice patterns emerging in your eating habits. Perhaps you tend to reach for sugary snacks when you're stressed, or you skip meals when you're busy and then overeat later in the day. Maybe you find yourself eating out of boredom or habit, rather than true hunger.

These patterns provide valuable clues about your relationship with food and can help you identify areas for improvement. By shining a light on these patterns, you can begin to make conscious choices that support your health and well-being, rather than undermine it.

Cultivating Mindful Eating

One of the key benefits of keeping a food diary is that it encourages mindful eating—the practice of being fully present and aware of your eating experience. By recording your meals and snacks in your food diary, you become more attuned to your body's hunger and satiety cues, allowing you to eat more intuitively and in line with your body's needs.

Mindful eating also helps to break the cycle of unconscious eating habits, such as eating in front of the TV or computer, or eating on the go without paying attention to what you're consuming. By bringing awareness to your eating habits, you can begin to savor and enjoy your food more fully, leading to greater satisfaction and fulfillment.

Evaluating Physical Activity Levels

Physical activity is not just about burning calories or sculpting our bodies—it's about supporting every aspect of our health, from cardiovascular health and bone density to mental well-being and cognitive function.

By assessing our physical activity levels, we gain valuable insight into how well we're meeting our bodies' needs for movement and exercise. This allows us to identify areas for improvement, set goals, and make informed choices that support our health and vitality.

Assessing Your Current Activity Levels

The first step in evaluating physical activity levels is to assess your current habits and routines. Take a moment to reflect on how much physical activity you engage in on a daily basis. Do you have a regular exercise routine, or do you lead a more sedentary lifestyle? How much time do you spend sitting, standing, walking, and engaging in structured exercise?

Be honest with yourself as you assess your current activity levels, and resist the temptation to judge or criticize. Remember, the purpose of assessment is not to place blame, but rather to gain insight and understanding into your habits and behaviors.

Understanding Different Types of Activity

Physical activity comes in many forms, and it's important to consider all aspects of movement when evaluating your activity levels. This includes structured exercise such as running, cycling, or strength training, as well as everyday activities such as walking, gardening, and household chores. It's also important to consider both aerobic exercise, which strengthens the heart and lungs, and resistance training, which builds muscle and bone strength. Each type of activity offers unique benefits and contributes to overall health and well-being.

Setting Goals for Improvement

Once you've assessed your current activity levels, it's time to set goals for improvement. Consider what areas of your physical activity routine could use some attention, and set specific, measurable goals to help you make progress.

For example, if you're currently leading a sedentary lifestyle, you might set a goal to incorporate more movement into your daily routine by taking regular breaks to stretch or go for short walks. If you're already active but looking to challenge yourself, you might set a goal to increase the intensity or duration of your workouts.

Identifying Habits Impacting Metabolism

Our habits play a starring role, shaping the way our bodies process energy and fuel our daily activities. But how often do we pause to consider the impact of our habits on our metabolic health? Join me as we delve into the practice of identifying habits impacting metabolism—a vital step towards optimizing our body's natural processes and unlocking our full potential for health and vitality.

Understanding Metabolism

Before we can delve into the habits impacting metabolism, it's important to have a basic understanding of what metabolism is and how it works.

At its core, metabolism refers to the complex series of chemical reactions that occur within our bodies to convert food into energy. This energy powers everything we do, from breathing and circulation to movement and exercise.

Our metabolic rate, or the speed at which our bodies burn calories, is influenced by a variety of factors, including genetics, age, gender, and body composition. But perhaps most importantly, our metabolism is influenced by our lifestyle habits—diet, exercise, sleep, stress management, and more—all of which play a significant role in determining how efficiently our bodies burn calories and process nutrients.

Assessing Your Habits

The first step in identifying habits impacting metabolism is to take a closer look at your daily routines and behaviors. Consider how you eat, move, sleep, and manage stress on a daily basis, and reflect on how these habits may be influencing your metabolic health.

For example, do you tend to skip meals or eat irregularly throughout the day? Do you rely heavily on processed foods and sugary snacks for energy? Are you getting enough physical activity and exercise, or do you lead a predominantly sedentary lifestyle? Do you prioritize sleep and relaxation, or do you often find yourself burning the candle at both ends?

Recognizing Habits That Support Metabolism

Once you've assessed your habits, it's time to identify those that support a healthy metabolism and promote optimal metabolic function. These habits are like fuel for your metabolic fire, providing the nutrients, energy, and support your body needs to thrive.

Healthy eating habits, such as consuming a balanced diet rich in fruits, vegetables, lean proteins, and whole grains, provide your body with the nutrients it needs to fuel metabolic processes and maintain energy levels throughout the day. Regular physical activity and exercise help to boost metabolism, build lean muscle mass, and improve insulin sensitivity, leading to more efficient calorie burning and nutrient utilization.

Adequate sleep and stress management are also crucial for supporting a healthy metabolism. Chronic stress and sleep deprivation can disrupt hormonal balance, increase cortisol levels, and interfere with metabolic function, leading to weight gain, insulin resistance, and other metabolic disorders.

Identifying Habits That Hinder Metabolism

In addition to recognizing habits that support metabolism, it's equally important to identify those that may be hindering your metabolic health. These habits act like roadblocks, impeding the body's ability to efficiently burn calories and process nutrients, and can have negative implications for overall health and well-being.

Poor dietary choices, such as excessive consumption of processed foods, sugary beverages, and unhealthy fats, can wreak havoc on metabolic health, leading to weight gain, inflammation, and insulin resistance. Sedentary behavior, such as prolonged sitting and lack of exercise, can slow metabolism and increase the risk of obesity, diabetes, and cardiovascular disease.

Chronic stress and sleep deprivation are also major culprits when it comes to sabotaging metabolism. Elevated cortisol levels and disrupted sleep patterns can lead to increased appetite, cravings for high-calorie foods, and impaired glucose metabolism, all of which can contribute to weight gain and metabolic dysfunction.

Making Positive Changes

Once you've identified habits impacting metabolism, the next step is to make positive changes that support your metabolic health and well-being. Start by focusing on small, manageable changes that you can incorporate into your daily routine, such as:

- Eating a balanced diet rich in whole, nutrient-dense foods
- Engaging in regular physical activity and exercise
- Prioritizing sleep and relaxation
- Managing stress through techniques such as mindfulness, meditation, and deep breathing exercises
- Avoiding excessive consumption of processed foods, sugary snacks, and unhealthy fats

THE SCIENCE BEHIND THE METABOLISM RESET DIET

Metabolism Basics: How Your Body Burns Calories

Metabolism serves as the conductor, orchestrating the complex symphony of chemical reactions that power our bodies and sustain life. But how exactly does metabolism work, and what role does it play in the process of burning calories? Join me as we delve into the fascinating world of metabolism basics and uncover the secrets of how your body burns calories.

The Metabolic Fire

At its core, metabolism refers to the sum total of all the chemical reactions that occur within the body to maintain life. This includes everything from digesting food and synthesizing nutrients to powering cellular activities and eliminating waste. In essence, metabolism is the engine that keeps our bodies running, providing the energy we need to carry out daily activities and functions.

But perhaps the most intriguing aspect of metabolism is its role in burning calories. Calories are a measure of energy, and the body relies on a continuous supply of calories to fuel its metabolic processes and support vital functions. When we talk about "burning calories," what we're really referring to is the process by which the body converts calories from food into energy that can be used to power our muscles, organs, and other tissues.

The Calorie Equation

The process of burning calories is governed by a simple yet elegant equation: calories in versus calories out. This equation represents the balance between the calories we consume through food and drink and the calories we expend through physical activity, exercise, and metabolic processes.

When we consume more calories than we expend, the excess calories are stored in the form of fat, leading to weight gain and potentially contributing to health problems such as obesity and metabolic syndrome. Conversely, when we expend more calories than we consume, the body must tap into its energy reserves to meet its needs, resulting in weight loss and improved metabolic health.

The Role of Basal Metabolic Rate

One of the key factors influencing how your body burns calories is your basal metabolic rate (BMR)—the amount of energy your body requires to maintain basic physiological functions while at rest. These functions include breathing, circulation, temperature regulation, and cell repair and maintenance.

Your BMR accounts for the majority of the calories you burn each day—up to 60-75% of total energy expenditure—making it a critical factor in determining overall metabolic rate and calorie burn. Factors that influence BMR include age, gender, body composition, and genetics, with lean muscle mass generally associated with higher metabolic rates due to its higher energy requirements.

The Thermic Effect of Food

In addition to basal metabolic rate, another factor that influences how your body burns calories is the thermic effect of food (TEF)—the energy expended by the body to digest, absorb, and metabolize nutrients from food. Different macronutrients have different TEF values, with protein requiring the most energy to digest (around 20-30% of total calories consumed), followed by carbohydrates (around 5-10%) and fats (around 0-3%).

By including a balance of protein, carbohydrates, and fats in your diet, you can maximize the thermic effect of food and enhance calorie burn. Additionally, spreading your meals and snacks throughout the day can help to keep your metabolism revved up and your energy levels stable, as the body expends energy to process and metabolize food.

The Role of Physical Activity

Of course, one of the most significant factors influencing how your body burns calories is physical activity and exercise. When you engage in physical activity, your muscles require energy to perform work, and the body must tap into its energy reserves to fuel this activity. This results in an increase in calorie burn, both during and after exercise, as the body works to replenish energy stores and repair muscle tissue.

The type, intensity, and duration of physical activity all play a role in determining calorie burn, with activities such as high-intensity interval training (HIIT) and strength training generally associated with higher calorie expenditure due to their greater metabolic demands. Additionally, incorporating more movement into your daily routine—such as walking, biking, or taking the stairs—can help to boost calorie burn and support overall metabolic health.

Hormonal Factors Affecting Metabolism in Endomorph Women

Hormones are powerful chemical messengers that regulate a wide range of bodily functions, including metabolism, growth, reproduction, and mood. In the context of metabolism, hormones play a central role in determining how efficiently the body burns calories, processes nutrients, and stores or utilizes energy.

For endomorph women, hormonal factors can have a significant impact on metabolic health and body composition, influencing everything from appetite and fat storage to energy levels and overall well-being. Understanding the interplay of hormones is essential for navigating the complexities of metabolism and achieving optimal health.

Estrogen and Progesterone

Two of the primary hormones that influence metabolism in endomorph women are estrogen and progesterone. Estrogen is known for its role in regulating the menstrual cycle, but it also plays a key role in metabolism by influencing fat distribution, insulin sensitivity, and energy expenditure.

Progesterone, on the other hand, works in tandem with estrogen to regulate the menstrual cycle and support reproductive health. It also has metabolic effects, such as increasing basal metabolic rate and promoting fat burning, which can help to offset some of the metabolic challenges associated with estrogen dominance.

Thyroid Hormones

The thyroid gland produces hormones that regulate metabolism, including thyroxine (T4) and triiodothyronine (T3). These hormones play a crucial role in determining the body's metabolic rate, controlling energy expenditure, and maintaining temperature regulation.

In endomorph women, thyroid function can be influenced by a variety of factors, including stress, nutrient deficiencies, and hormonal imbalances. Hypothyroidism, or underactive thyroid function, can lead to a slowing of metabolism and weight gain, while hyperthyroidism, or overactive thyroid function, can result in an increase in metabolism and unintended weight loss.

Insulin and Glucagon

Insulin and glucagon are hormones that regulate blood sugar levels and play a key role in metabolism. Insulin helps to transport glucose from the bloodstream into cells, where it can be used for energy or stored as glycogen or fat. Glucagon, on the other hand, works to raise blood sugar levels by promoting the breakdown of glycogen into glucose and stimulating gluconeogenesis, the production of glucose from non-carbohydrate sources.

In endomorph women, hormonal imbalances such as insulin resistance can disrupt the delicate balance between insulin and glucagon, leading to dysregulation of blood sugar levels and impaired metabolism. This can contribute to weight gain, increased fat storage, and a host of metabolic health issues.

Cortisol and Stress Hormones

Cortisol, often referred to as the "stress hormone," plays a critical role in the body's response to stress and helps to regulate metabolism, immune function, and inflammation. In times of acute stress, cortisol levels rise, mobilizing energy stores and increasing metabolism to help the body cope with the demands of the situation.

However, chronic stress and elevated cortisol levels can have detrimental effects on metabolism, leading to increased appetite, cravings for high-calorie foods, and abdominal fat accumulation. This can create a vicious cycle of stress and weight gain, further exacerbating metabolic health issues in endomorph women.

Strategies for Optimizing Metabolic Rate

Metabolic rate, often referred to as metabolism, is the amount of energy (calories) your body expends to maintain basic physiological functions while at rest. This includes activities such as breathing, circulation, temperature regulation, and cell repair and maintenance. In essence, metabolic rate represents the total energy expenditure of your body at rest, expressed in calories per day.

Several factors influence metabolic rate, including age, gender, body composition, genetics, and hormonal factors. For example, lean muscle mass is associated with a higher metabolic rate due to its higher energy requirements, while age-related changes and hormonal imbalances can lead to declines in metabolic rate over time.

Optimizing Nutritional Intake

One of the most effective strategies for optimizing metabolic rate is to focus on your nutritional intake. By fueling your body with the right nutrients in the right proportions, you can support metabolic function and enhance calorie burn.

- **Balanced Diet**: Aim for a balanced diet rich in whole, nutrient-dense foods such as fruits, vegetables, lean proteins, and whole grains. These foods provide the vitamins, minerals, and macronutrients your body needs to fuel metabolic processes and maintain energy levels.

- **Protein Intake**: Protein plays a key role in metabolism, as it requires more energy to digest and metabolize compared to carbohydrates and fats. Aim to include lean sources of protein such as chicken, fish, tofu, and legumes in your meals and snacks to support muscle growth, repair, and maintenance.

- **Hydration**: Staying hydrated is essential for optimal metabolic function. Water plays a crucial role in numerous metabolic processes, including nutrient transport, temperature regulation, and waste elimination. Aim to drink plenty of water throughout the day to support hydration and metabolic health.

Incorporating Physical Activity

Physical activity is another critical factor in optimizing metabolic rate. Regular exercise not only burns calories during the activity itself but also increases metabolic rate for hours afterward, leading to greater calorie burn and metabolic efficiency over time.

- **Strength Training**: Incorporate strength training exercises into your workout routine to build lean muscle mass and boost metabolic rate. Muscle tissue is more metabolically active than fat tissue, meaning that the more muscle you have, the more calories you burn at rest.

- **Cardiovascular Exercise**: Cardiovascular exercise, such as running, cycling, or swimming, is also effective for boosting metabolic rate and burning calories. Aim for at least 150 minutes of moderate-intensity aerobic activity or 75 minutes of vigorous-intensity activity per week to support metabolic health.

- **High-Intensity Interval Training (HIIT)**: HIIT workouts involve alternating between short bursts of intense exercise and brief periods of rest or recovery. This type of training has been shown to increase metabolic rate and calorie burn both during and after exercise, making it an efficient and effective way to optimize metabolic health.

Prioritizing Sleep and Stress Management

Finally, prioritizing sleep and stress management is essential for optimizing metabolic rate and overall well-being. Chronic stress and sleep deprivation can disrupt hormonal balance, increase cortisol levels, and impair metabolic function, leading to weight gain, insulin resistance, and other metabolic health issues.

- **Quality Sleep**: Aim for 7-9 hours of quality sleep per night to support hormonal balance, metabolic function, and overall health. Create a relaxing bedtime routine, limit exposure to screens and electronic devices before bed, and create a comfortable sleep environment to promote restful sleep.

- **Stress Management**: Incorporate stress-reducing activities such as meditation, deep breathing exercises, yoga, or tai chi into your daily routine to promote relaxation and reduce stress levels. Practice mindfulness and self-care to cultivate a sense of balance and well-being in your life.

ESSENTIAL NUTRIENTS FOR ENDOMORPHS

Macronutrient Balance: Protein, Carbohydrates, and Fats

Macronutrients serve as the building blocks of life, providing the energy and nutrients our bodies need to thrive. But how exactly do these macronutrients—protein, carbohydrates, and fats—work together to support our health and well-being? Join me as we explore the fascinating world of macronutrient balance and uncover the secrets to optimizing your diet for optimal health.

The Role of Protein

Protein is often hailed as the king of macronutrients, and for good reason. It serves as the foundation for building and repairing tissues, including muscles, bones, skin, and hair. Additionally, protein plays a crucial role in supporting immune function, hormone production, and enzyme activity throughout the body.

When it comes to macronutrient balance, protein is essential for maintaining muscle mass, supporting weight management, and promoting satiety and fullness. Including a source of protein in each meal and snack can help to stabilize blood sugar levels, prevent overeating, and support overall metabolic health.

Choosing High-Quality Protein Sources

Not all proteins are created equal, and choosing high-quality sources of protein is essential for maximizing the health benefits of this macronutrient. Aim to include a variety of protein-rich foods in your diet, such as:

- Lean meats such as chicken, turkey, and fish
- Eggs and dairy products such as Greek yogurt and cottage cheese
- Plant-based sources such as tofu, tempeh, legumes, and quinoa

By incorporating a variety of protein sources into your diet, you can ensure that you're getting all the essential amino acids your body needs to support optimal health and vitality.

The Role of Carbohydrates

Carbohydrates are often vilified in the world of nutrition, but the truth is, they play a crucial role in supporting energy production, brain function, and overall metabolic health. Carbohydrates are the body's preferred source of fuel, providing the energy needed to power our daily activities and functions.

When it comes to macronutrient balance, carbohydrates are essential for supporting physical activity, replenishing glycogen stores, and maintaining blood sugar levels. Including a mix of complex carbohydrates such as whole grains, fruits, vegetables, and legumes in your diet can help to provide sustained energy and support overall health and well-being.

Choosing Healthy Carbohydrate Sources

Not all carbohydrates are created equal, and choosing healthy sources of carbohydrates is key for supporting metabolic health and overall well-being. Aim to focus on whole, minimally processed carbohydrates that are rich in fiber, vitamins, and minerals, such as:

- Whole grains such as brown rice, quinoa, oats, and barley
- Fruits and vegetables such as berries, apples, leafy greens, and sweet potatoes

- Legumes such as beans, lentils, and chickpeas

By choosing these nutrient-dense carbohydrate sources, you can fuel your body with the energy it needs to thrive while supporting overall health and vitality.

The Role of Fats

Fats often get a bad rap, but the truth is, they're an essential part of a healthy diet. Fats play a crucial role in supporting cell structure, hormone production, brain function, and nutrient absorption. Additionally, dietary fats provide a concentrated source of energy, helping to fuel our bodies during times of rest and activity.

When it comes to macronutrient balance, including healthy fats in your diet is essential for supporting satiety, promoting heart health, and maintaining metabolic function. Aim to include a mix of unsaturated fats such as:

- Avocados
- Nuts and seeds
- Olive oil
- Fatty fish such as salmon, mackerel, and sardines

These healthy fats not only provide essential nutrients and energy but also help to support overall health and well-being.

Finding the Right Balance

Achieving macronutrient balance is all about finding the right mix of protein, carbohydrates, and fats that works best for your body and lifestyle. Experiment with different foods and meal combinations to find what feels best for you, and don't be afraid to adjust your macronutrient intake based on your individual needs and goals.

Remember, there's no one-size-fits-all approach to nutrition, and what works for one person may not work for another. Listen to your body, pay attention to how different foods make you feel, and prioritize nutrient-dense whole foods to support your health and well-being.

Micronutrients for Energy Production and Hormonal Balance

Micronutrients serve as the unsung heroes, playing a vital role in supporting energy production, hormone regulation, and overall metabolic function. But what exactly are micronutrients, and how do they contribute to our energy levels and hormonal balance? Join me as we explore the fascinating world of micronutrients and uncover the secrets to optimizing your diet for vitality and well-being.

Understanding Micronutrients

Micronutrients are essential vitamins and minerals that the body requires in small amounts to function properly. These micronutrients play a variety of roles in the body, including supporting metabolism, promoting cellular energy production, and regulating hormone levels. While they may be needed in smaller quantities compared to macronutrients, their importance cannot be overstated when it comes to overall health and well-being.

Vitamins for Energy Production

Several vitamins play a crucial role in energy production and metabolism, helping to convert food into usable energy for the body. Some of the key vitamins involved in this process include:

- **B Vitamins**: The B-complex vitamins, including B1 (thiamine), B2 (riboflavin), B3 (niacin), B5 (pantothenic acid), B6 (pyridoxine), B7 (biotin), B9 (folate), and B12 (cobalamin), are essential for converting carbohydrates, fats, and proteins into energy. They also play a role in supporting nervous system function and red blood cell production.

- **Vitamin C**: Vitamin C is an antioxidant vitamin that plays a key role in energy metabolism, supporting the synthesis of carnitine, a molecule that helps transport fatty acids into the mitochondria for energy production. Additionally, vitamin C is involved in collagen synthesis, immune function, and wound healing.

- **Vitamin D**: While primarily known for its role in calcium absorption and bone health, vitamin D also plays a role in energy metabolism, muscle function, and immune regulation. Low levels of vitamin D have been associated with fatigue and decreased energy levels, highlighting the importance of adequate vitamin D intake for overall well-being.

Minerals for Hormonal Balance

In addition to vitamins, minerals also play a crucial role in supporting hormonal balance and metabolic function. These minerals act as cofactors for enzymes involved in hormone synthesis, transport, and receptor function, helping to regulate hormone levels and promote overall health and vitality. Some of the key minerals involved in hormonal balance include:

- **Magnesium**: Magnesium plays a crucial role in over 300 enzymatic reactions in the body, including those involved in energy metabolism, muscle function, and hormone regulation. It helps to support insulin sensitivity, cortisol regulation, and thyroid function, making it essential for overall metabolic health.

- **Zinc**: Zinc is involved in numerous processes in the body, including immune function, wound healing, and DNA synthesis. It also plays a role in hormone production and regulation, particularly testosterone and thyroid hormones. Low levels of zinc have been associated with hormonal imbalances and metabolic dysfunction, highlighting the importance of adequate zinc intake for overall health.

- **Iron**: Iron is essential for the production of hemoglobin, a protein in red blood cells that carries oxygen from the lungs to the tissues. It also plays a role in energy metabolism, supporting cellular energy production and overall metabolic function. Iron deficiency can lead to fatigue, weakness, and decreased energy levels, underscoring the importance of adequate iron intake for overall well-being.

Incorporating Micronutrients into Your Diet

Now that we understand the importance of micronutrients for energy production and hormonal balance, the next question is: how can we ensure we're getting enough of these vital nutrients in our diet? The answer lies in eating a diverse and nutrient-rich diet that includes a variety of fruits, vegetables, whole grains, lean proteins, and healthy fats.

- **Colorful Fruits and Vegetables**: Aim to fill your plate with a rainbow of colorful fruits and vegetables, as these foods are rich in vitamins, minerals, and antioxidants that support overall health and well-being. Include a mix of leafy greens, berries, citrus fruits, cruciferous vegetables, and root vegetables to ensure you're getting a wide range of micronutrients.

- **Lean Proteins**: Incorporate lean sources of protein into your diet, such as poultry, fish, tofu, tempeh, legumes, and low-fat dairy products. These foods not only provide essential amino acids for muscle repair and growth but also contain micronutrients such as B vitamins, iron, and zinc that support energy production and hormonal balance.

- **Whole Grains**: Choose whole grains such as brown rice, quinoa, oats, barley, and whole wheat bread and pasta over refined grains to ensure you're getting the full spectrum of nutrients and fiber. Whole grains provide complex carbohydrates for sustained energy, along with vitamins, minerals, and antioxidants that support overall health and well-being.

Hydration and Its Role in Metabolism

Hydration is the process of replenishing the body's fluid levels to maintain optimal function of cells, tissues, and organs. Water, the elixir of life, serves as the primary component of hydration, accounting for approximately 60% of the human body's total weight. Adequate hydration is essential for numerous physiological processes, including temperature regulation, nutrient transport, waste removal, and metabolic function.

The Role of Water in Metabolism

Water plays a crucial role in metabolism, serving as a key component of various metabolic processes that occur within the body. These processes include:

- **Digestion and Absorption**: Water is essential for breaking down food particles and facilitating the absorption of nutrients in the gastrointestinal tract. It helps to dissolve nutrients, enzymes, and other digestive secretions, allowing them to be transported across the intestinal lining and into the bloodstream for use by the body.

- **Nutrient Transport**: Once absorbed, nutrients are transported throughout the body via the bloodstream, where they are delivered to cells and tissues to support various metabolic functions. Water helps to maintain blood volume and circulation, ensuring that nutrients reach their intended destinations and metabolic processes can proceed efficiently.

- **Energy Production**: Water is involved in the production of energy within cells through a process known as cellular respiration. During cellular respiration, glucose and oxygen are metabolized to produce ATP (adenosine triphosphate), the primary energy currency of the body. Water molecules are used as reactants and byproducts in this process, making hydration essential for energy production.

- **Temperature Regulation**: Water plays a crucial role in regulating body temperature through processes such as sweating and evaporation. During physical activity or exposure to high temperatures, the body loses water through sweat, which helps to dissipate heat and cool the body down. Adequate hydration is essential for maintaining optimal body temperature and preventing dehydration and overheating.

The Impact of Dehydration on Metabolism

Dehydration occurs when the body loses more fluid than it takes in, leading to an imbalance in fluid levels and impairments in metabolic function. Even mild dehydration can have profound effects on metabolism, including:

- **Slowed Metabolic Rate**: Dehydration can lead to a decrease in metabolic rate, as the body conserves energy and prioritizes essential functions to maintain hydration and fluid balance. This can result in decreased calorie burn and reduced energy levels, making it more difficult to maintain weight or achieve weight loss goals.

- **Impaired Nutrient Absorption**: Dehydration can impair the absorption of nutrients in the gastrointestinal tract, leading to deficiencies in essential vitamins and minerals that are necessary for metabolic function. This can hinder energy production, nutrient metabolism, and overall metabolic health.

- **Increased Fatigue and Decreased Performance**: Dehydration can lead to increased fatigue, decreased cognitive function, and impaired physical performance, making it more difficult to engage in physical activity or exercise. This can further exacerbate metabolic imbalances and hinder progress towards health and fitness goals.

Strategies for Optimal Hydration

Ensuring adequate hydration is essential for supporting metabolism and overall health and well-being. Here are some strategies to help you stay hydrated and optimize your metabolic function:

- **Drink Plenty of Water**: Aim to drink at least 8-10 cups of water per day, or more if you're physically active or exposed to hot temperatures. Carry a reusable water bottle with you throughout the day as a reminder to stay hydrated, and sip water regularly to maintain fluid balance.

- **Eat Hydrating Foods**: Incorporate hydrating foods into your diet, such as fruits and vegetables with high water content. Cucumber, watermelon, strawberries, oranges, and celery are all excellent choices that can help contribute to your daily fluid intake.

- **Monitor Your Urine Color**: Pay attention to the color of your urine as a simple indicator of hydration status. Pale yellow or straw-colored urine indicates adequate hydration, while darker urine may indicate dehydration and the need to drink more fluids.

- **Listen to Your Body**: Tune in to your body's thirst signals and drink water whenever you feel thirsty. Thirst is a natural mechanism that signals the body's need for fluid replenishment, so be sure to respond promptly to maintain hydration and support metabolic function.

CREATING YOUR MEAL PLAN

Designing a Balanced Meal Plan for Endomorphs

For endomorphs, individuals with a predisposition to store fat and a slower metabolic rate, the importance of a balanced meal plan cannot be overstated. But what exactly does a balanced meal plan look like for endomorphs, and how can it support their unique metabolic needs? Join me as we explore the art of crafting a meal plan that nourishes both body and soul, empowering endomorphs to thrive in their journey towards health and vitality.

Understanding the Endomorphic Body

Endomorphs are characterized by a tendency to store excess fat, particularly in the midsection, hips, and thighs. They typically have a slower metabolic rate and may struggle with weight management and maintaining lean muscle mass. While genetics play a significant role in determining body type, lifestyle factors such as diet and exercise also play a crucial role in shaping body composition and overall health.

Key Principles of a Balanced Meal Plan for Endomorphs

A balanced meal plan for endomorphs should focus on:

- **Balanced Macronutrient Ratio**: Endomorphs may benefit from a meal plan that includes a balanced ratio of macronutrients, including protein, carbohydrates, and fats. Aim to include lean sources of protein, complex carbohydrates, and healthy fats in each meal to support satiety, stabilize blood sugar levels, and promote overall metabolic health.

- **Portion Control**: Endomorphs may be more prone to overeating, so portion control is key to managing calorie intake and supporting weight management goals. Focus on mindful eating practices, such as eating slowly, paying attention to hunger and fullness cues, and avoiding distractions during meals.

- **Fiber-Rich Foods**: Including fiber-rich foods such as fruits, vegetables, whole grains, and legumes in your meal plan can help to promote feelings of fullness, support digestive health, and regulate blood sugar levels. Aim to include a variety of colorful fruits and vegetables in your meals to ensure you're getting a wide range of nutrients and fiber.

- **Hydration**: Adequate hydration is essential for supporting metabolic function, promoting satiety, and maintaining overall health and well-being. Aim to drink plenty of water throughout the day and incorporate hydrating foods such as fruits and vegetables into your meal plan to support hydration and overall health.

Sample Meal Plan for Endomorphs

Here's a sample meal plan that incorporates the key principles outlined above:

- **Breakfast**: Scrambled eggs with spinach and tomatoes, whole grain toast, and avocado slices

- **Mid-Morning Snack**: Greek yogurt with berries and a handful of almonds

- **Lunch**: Grilled chicken salad with mixed greens, cucumber, bell peppers, and quinoa, dressed with olive oil and balsamic vinegar

- **Afternoon Snack**: Carrot sticks with hummus

- **Dinner**: Baked salmon with roasted sweet potatoes and steamed broccoli

- **Evening Snack**: Apple slices with almond butter

Tips for Success

- **Plan Ahead**: Take the time to plan your meals and snacks for the week ahead, and stock your kitchen with nutritious ingredients to make meal prep a breeze.

- **Listen to Your Body**: Pay attention to how different foods make you feel, and adjust your meal plan accordingly to support your energy levels, digestion, and overall well-being.

- **Stay Consistent**: Consistency is key to success when it comes to nutrition and health. Stick to your meal plan as much as possible, but don't be too hard on yourself if you stray from time to time. Remember, it's about progress, not perfection.

Portion Control Strategies for Weight Management

Portion control stands as a powerful tool in our arsenal, allowing us to navigate the sea of temptation and achieve our health and wellness goals. But what exactly is portion control, and how can it empower us on our journey towards a healthier, happier self? Join me as we delve into the art of portion control and uncover strategies to help you take control of your eating habits and achieve lasting success in your weight management journey.

Understanding Portion Control

Portion control is the practice of managing the quantity of food we consume during meals and snacks to regulate calorie intake and support weight management goals. It involves being mindful of portion sizes and making conscious choices about how much food we eat, rather than relying on external cues or habits to determine our intake. By practicing portion control, we can prevent overeating, regulate hunger and fullness cues, and maintain a healthy balance between energy intake and expenditure.

Portion Control Strategies

Here are some effective strategies to help you master portion control and achieve success in your weight management journey:

1. Use Visual Cues

Visual cues can be powerful tools for gauging portion sizes and preventing overeating. Try using your hand as a guide for portion sizes:

- **Protein**: Aim for a palm-sized portion of protein, such as chicken, fish, tofu, or lean meat.

- **Carbohydrates**: Limit carbohydrate servings to about the size of your clenched fist, whether it's rice, pasta, or potatoes.

- **Vegetables**: Load up on non-starchy vegetables, aiming for at least two handfuls per meal.

- **Fats**: Limit healthy fats like nuts, seeds, or avocado to the size of your thumb.

2. Practice Mindful Eating

Mindful eating involves paying attention to the sensory experience of eating, including the taste, texture, and aroma of food, as well as hunger and fullness cues. By slowing down and savoring each bite, you can become more attuned to your body's signals of hunger and fullness, helping you to avoid overeating and make healthier choices.

3. Use Smaller Plates and Bowls

The size of our plates and bowls can influence our perception of portion sizes and affect how much we eat. Using smaller plates and bowls can trick our brains into thinking we're eating more than we actually are, helping to reduce portion sizes and prevent overeating. Opt for salad plates or smaller bowls to help control portion sizes and promote mindful eating.

4. Pre-Portion Snacks and Treats

Pre-portioning snacks and treats into individual servings can help prevent mindless munching and overeating. Instead of eating straight from the bag or container, portion out servings into small bags or containers ahead of time. This can help you stick to appropriate portion sizes and avoid the temptation to eat more than you intended.

5. Listen to Your Body

Pay attention to your body's hunger and fullness cues, and eat only when you're truly hungry. Avoid eating out of boredom, stress, or habit, and tune in to how different foods make you feel. Stop eating when you feel satisfied, rather than waiting until you're uncomfortably full, and be mindful of emotional eating triggers.

Incorporating Portion Control into Your Lifestyle

By incorporating these portion control strategies into your daily routine, you can take control of your eating habits and achieve lasting success in your weight management journey. Remember, portion control is not about deprivation or restriction, but rather about making conscious choices that support your health and well-being. With practice and patience, you can learn to enjoy food in moderation and achieve balance in your eating habits.

Incorporating Whole Foods and Nutrient-Dense Ingredients

Whole foods and nutrient-dense ingredients stand as the vibrant threads that weave together a tapestry of health and vitality. But what exactly are whole foods, and why are they so important for our well-being? Join me as we explore the world of whole foods and nutrient-dense ingredients, and discover how they can nourish your body from the inside out.

Understanding Whole Foods

Whole foods are foods that are minimally processed and close to their natural state, as they are found in nature. These foods are rich in nutrients, including vitamins, minerals, fiber, and antioxidants, and provide essential nourishment for our bodies. Examples of whole foods include fruits, vegetables, whole grains, legumes, nuts, seeds, and lean proteins such as poultry, fish, and tofu.

The Importance of Whole Foods

Incorporating whole foods into your diet offers a multitude of health benefits, including:

- **Nutrient Density**: Whole foods are packed with essential nutrients that are vital for optimal health and well-being. By choosing whole foods over processed alternatives, you can ensure that your body receives the vitamins, minerals, and antioxidants it needs to function at its best.

- **Fiber Content**: Whole foods are rich in dietary fiber, which plays a crucial role in digestive health, weight management, and disease prevention. Fiber helps to regulate bowel movements, promote satiety, and stabilize blood sugar levels, making it an essential component of a healthy diet.

- **Antioxidant Power**: Many whole foods are rich in antioxidants, which help to protect our cells from damage caused by free radicals and oxidative stress. Antioxidants have been linked to a reduced risk of chronic diseases such as heart disease, cancer, and neurodegenerative disorders, making them an important part of a healthy diet.

Incorporating Whole Foods into Your Diet

Here are some tips for incorporating more whole foods into your diet and reaping the benefits of their nutritional goodness:

1. Shop the Perimeter of the Grocery Store

The perimeter of the grocery store is where you'll find the majority of whole foods, including fresh produce, lean proteins, dairy products, and whole grains. By focusing your shopping efforts on the perimeter, you can avoid the processed and packaged foods that often line the aisles and make healthier choices for you and your family.

2. Fill Your Plate with Color

When planning your meals, aim to fill your plate with a rainbow of colors by including a variety of fruits and vegetables in your diet. Different colored fruits and vegetables contain different vitamins, minerals, and antioxidants, so incorporating a diverse range of colors into your meals ensures that you're getting a wide range of nutrients to support your health.

3. Choose Whole Grains

Swap refined grains for whole grains such as brown rice, quinoa, oats, and whole wheat bread and pasta. Whole grains are higher in fiber and nutrients than their refined counterparts and can help to promote satiety, stabilize blood sugar levels, and support digestive health.

4. Snack Smart

Opt for nutrient-dense snacks such as fresh fruit, raw vegetables, nuts, seeds, and yogurt instead of processed snacks like chips, cookies, and candy. These whole food snacks provide a satisfying combination of vitamins, minerals, fiber, and protein to keep you feeling full and satisfied between meals.

5. Get Creative in the Kitchen

Experiment with new recipes and cooking techniques to incorporate more whole foods into your meals. Try roasting vegetables, blending smoothies, or making homemade soups and salads using fresh, seasonal ingredients. Get creative with herbs, spices, and healthy fats like olive oil and avocado to add flavor and variety to your meals.

BREAKFAST RECIPES

Protein-Packed Breakfast Burrito

Prep Time: 15 mins

Total Time: 20 mins

Servings: 2

Ingredients:

- 4 large eggs
- ½ cup black beans, drained and rinsed
- ½ cup diced tomatoes
- ¼ cup diced bell peppers
- ¼ cup diced onions
- ½ avocado, sliced
- 2 whole grain tortillas
- Salt and pepper to taste
- Optional: salsa, Greek yogurt, shredded cheese

Directions:

1. In a bowl, whisk together the eggs and season with salt and pepper.
2. In a skillet over medium heat, add the eggs and scramble until cooked through.
3. Warm the tortillas in the skillet or microwave.
4. Assemble the burritos by dividing the scrambled eggs, black beans, tomatoes, bell peppers, onions, and avocado between the tortillas.
5. Roll up the tortillas, tucking in the sides as you go.
6. Serve with salsa, Greek yogurt, or shredded cheese if desired.

Nutrition Facts (per serving):

- Calories: 380
- Fat: 18g
- Saturated fat: 4g
- Cholesterol: 370mg
- Sodium: 430mg
- Carbohydrate: 36g
- Fiber: 10g
- Protein: 21g
- Calcium: 150mg
- Iron: 4.5mg

Greek Yogurt Parfait

Prep Time: 5 mins

Total Time: 5 mins

Servings: 1

Ingredients:

- 1 cup Greek yogurt
- ½ cup mixed berries (strawberries, blueberries, raspberries)
- ¼ cup granola
- 1 tablespoon honey or maple syrup (optional)

Directions:

1. In a glass or bowl, layer Greek yogurt, mixed berries, and granola.
2. Drizzle with honey or maple syrup if desired.

Nutrition Facts (per serving):

- Calories: 320
- Fat: 7g

- Saturated fat: 1g

- Cholesterol: 10mg

- Sodium: 90mg

- Carbohydrate: 46g

- Fiber: 6g

- Sugar: 24g

- Protein: 22g

- Calcium: 240mg

- Iron: 1mg

Veggie Omelette

Prep Time: 10 mins

Total Time: 20 mins

Servings: 1

Ingredients:

- 2 large eggs

- ¼ cup diced bell peppers

- ¼ cup diced onions

- ¼ cup diced tomatoes

- ¼ cup spinach leaves

- Salt and pepper to taste

- 1 teaspoon olive oil

Directions:

1. In a bowl, whisk together the eggs and season with salt and pepper.

2. Heat olive oil in a skillet over medium heat.

3. Add bell peppers, onions, and tomatoes to the skillet and cook until softened.

4. Add spinach leaves to the skillet and cook until wilted.

5. Pour the whisked eggs into the skillet and cook until set.

6. Fold the omelette in half and serve hot.

Nutrition Facts (per serving):

- Calories: 220

- Fat: 14g

- Saturated fat: 3g

- Cholesterol: 370mg

- Sodium: 220mg

- Carbohydrate: 10g

- Fiber: 3g

- Sugar: 5g

- Protein: 16g

- Vitamin A: 40%

- Vitamin C: 60%

- Calcium: 6%

- Iron: 10%

Quinoa Breakfast Bowl

Prep Time: 5 mins

Total Time: 20 mins

Servings: 2

Ingredients:

- 1 cup cooked quinoa

- ½ cup sliced strawberries

- ½ cup blueberries

- ¼ cup chopped almonds

- 2 tablespoons honey or maple syrup

- ½ teaspoon cinnamon

Directions:

1. In a bowl, combine cooked quinoa, sliced strawberries, blueberries, and chopped almonds.

2. Drizzle with honey or maple syrup and sprinkle with cinnamon.

3. Stir to combine and serve warm or chilled.

Nutrition Facts (per serving):

- Calories: 320
- Fat: 10g
- Saturated fat: 1g
- Cholesterol: 0mg
- Sodium: 5mg
- Carbohydrate: 55g
- Fiber: 8g
- Sugar: 20g
- Protein: 9g
- Calcium: 90mg
- Iron: 2mg

Avocado Toast with Poached Egg

Prep Time: 10 mins

Total Time: 15 mins

Servings: 1

Ingredients:

- 1 slice whole grain bread, toasted
- ½ avocado, mashed
- 1 large egg

- Salt and pepper to taste
- Optional toppings: sliced tomatoes, microgreens, hot sauce

Directions:

1. Toast the whole grain bread until golden brown.
2. Spread mashed avocado on the toast and season with salt and pepper.
3. Poach the egg in simmering water until cooked to your desired doneness.
4. Place the poached egg on top of the avocado toast.
5. Add optional toppings such as sliced tomatoes, microgreens, or hot sauce if desired.

Nutrition Facts (per serving):

- Calories: 280
- Fat: 15g
- Saturated fat: 2.5g
- Cholesterol: 185mg
- Sodium: 190mg
- Carbohydrate: 26g
- Fiber: 7g
- Sugar: 1g
- Protein: 12g
- Vitamin D: 15%
- Calcium: 4%
- Iron: 10%
- Potassium: 590mg

Berry Blast Smoothie Bowl

Prep Time: 5 mins

Total Time: 5 mins

Servings: 1

Ingredients:

- 1 frozen banana
- ½ cup frozen mixed berries (strawberries, blueberries, raspberries)
- ½ cup spinach leaves
- ½ cup almond milk
- 1 tablespoon chia seeds
- Optional toppings: sliced banana, granola, shredded coconut

Directions:

1. In a blender, combine the frozen banana, frozen mixed berries, spinach leaves, almond milk, and chia seeds.
2. Blend until smooth and creamy, adding more almond milk if needed to reach desired consistency.
3. Pour the smoothie into a bowl and top with sliced banana, granola, and shredded coconut if desired.

Nutrition Facts (per serving):

- Calories: 280
- Fat: 9g
- Saturated fat: 1g
- Cholesterol: 0mg
- Sodium: 120mg
- Carbohydrate: 46g
- Fiber: 12g

- Sugar: 20g
- Protein: 7g
- Vitamin A: 60%
- Vitamin C: 80%
- Calcium: 35%
- Iron: 2mg

Veggie Egg Muffins

Prep Time: 10 mins

Total Time: 25 mins

Servings: 6

Ingredients:

- 6 large eggs
- ½ cup diced bell peppers
- ½ cup diced onions
- ½ cup diced tomatoes
- ½ cup spinach leaves
- Salt and pepper to taste
- Optional: shredded cheese

Directions:

1. Preheat the oven to 350°F (175°C) and grease a muffin tin.
2. In a bowl, whisk together the eggs and season with salt and pepper.
3. Stir in the diced bell peppers, onions, tomatoes, and spinach leaves.
4. Pour the egg mixture into the muffin tin, filling each cup about ¾ full.
5. If desired, sprinkle shredded cheese on top of each muffin.

6. Bake for 20-25 minutes, or until the egg muffins are set and lightly golden.

7. Allow to cool slightly before serving.

Nutrition Facts (per serving):

- Calories: 120
- Fat: 7g
- Saturated fat: 2g
- Cholesterol: 185mg
- Sodium: 120mg
- Carbohydrate: 5g
- Fiber: 1g
- Sugar: 2g
- Protein: 9g
- Vitamin A: 20%
- Vitamin C: 30%
- Calcium: 4%
- Iron: 1mg

Chia Seed Pudding

Prep Time: 5 mins

Total Time: 4 hours 5 mins

Servings: 2

Ingredients:

- ½ cup chia seeds
- 2 cups almond milk
- 1 tablespoon honey or maple syrup
- ½ teaspoon vanilla extract
- Optional toppings: sliced banana, berries, nuts, seeds

Directions:

1. In a bowl, combine chia seeds, almond milk, honey or maple syrup, and vanilla extract.
2. Whisk together until well combined.
3. Cover and refrigerate for at least 4 hours or overnight, stirring occasionally, until thickened.
4. Serve chilled with your choice of toppings.

Nutrition Facts (per serving):

- Calories: 210
- Fat: 11g
- Saturated fat: 1g
- Cholesterol: 0mg
- Sodium: 100mg
- Carbohydrate: 22g
- Fiber: 14g
- Sugar: 6g
- Protein: 7g
- Calcium: 40%
- Iron: 3mg

Spinach and Mushroom Breakfast Quesadilla

Prep Time: 10 mins

Total Time: 15 mins

Servings: 1

Ingredients:

- 1 whole grain tortilla
- 1 large egg
- ½ cup fresh spinach leaves

- ¼ cup sliced mushrooms
- 2 tablespoons shredded cheese
- Salt and pepper to taste
- Optional: salsa, Greek yogurt

Directions:

1. In a skillet over medium heat, cook the egg to your desired doneness (scrambled, fried, or poached).
2. Remove the egg from the skillet and set aside.
3. In the same skillet, add the spinach leaves and sliced mushrooms.
4. Cook until the spinach wilts and the mushrooms are tender.
5. Place the tortilla in the skillet and sprinkle with shredded cheese.
6. Top with the cooked egg, spinach, and mushrooms.
7. Fold the tortilla in half and cook until golden brown on both sides.
8. Serve hot with salsa and Greek yogurt if desired.

Nutrition Facts (per serving):

- Calories: 320
- Fat: 15g
- Saturated fat: 5g
- Cholesterol: 220mg
- Sodium: 520mg
- Carbohydrate: 25g
- Fiber: 5g
- Sugar: 1g
- Protein: 21g

- Vitamin A: 80%

- Vitamin C: 10%

- Calcium: 25%

- Iron: 3mg

Overnight Oats

Prep Time: 5 mins

Total Time: 8 hours 5 mins (overnight)

Servings: 1

Ingredients:

- ½ cup rolled oats

- ½ cup almond milk

- ½ cup Greek yogurt

- 1 tablespoon chia seeds

- 1 tablespoon honey or maple syrup

- ¼ teaspoon vanilla extract

- Optional toppings: sliced banana, berries, nuts, seeds

Directions:

1. In a jar or container, combine rolled oats, almond milk, Greek yogurt, chia seeds, honey or maple syrup, and vanilla extract.

2. Stir until well combined.

3. Cover and refrigerate overnight, or for at least 8 hours.

4. Stir well before serving and add your choice of toppings.

Nutrition Facts (per serving):

- Calories: 320

- Fat: 7g

- Saturated fat: 1g

- Cholesterol: 5mg

- Sodium: 120mg

- Carbohydrate: 52g

- Fiber: 8g

- Sugar: 18g

- Protein: 15g

- Calcium: 25%

- Iron: 2mg

Sweet Potato and Spinach Breakfast Hash

Prep Time: 10 mins

Total Time: 25 mins

Servings: 2

Ingredients: 1 large sweet potato, peeled and diced

- 2 cups fresh spinach leaves

- 1 bell pepper, diced

- ½ onion, diced

- 2 cloves garlic, minced

- 2 large eggs

- 2 tablespoons olive oil

- Salt and pepper to taste

- Optional toppings: sliced avocado, hot sauce

Directions:

1. Heat olive oil in a skillet over medium heat. Add the diced sweet potato and cook until tender and lightly browned, about 10-12 minutes.

2. Add the diced bell pepper, onion, and minced garlic to the skillet. Cook until the vegetables are softened.

3. Stir in the fresh spinach leaves and cook until wilted.

4. Create two wells in the hash and crack an egg into each well. Cook until the egg whites are set but the yolks are still runny.

5. Season with salt and pepper to taste.

6. Serve hot with optional toppings like sliced avocado or hot sauce.

Nutrition Facts (per serving):

- Calories: 300
- Fat: 15g
- Saturated fat: 3g
- Cholesterol: 185mg
- Sodium: 120mg
- Carbohydrate: 35g
- Fiber: 7g
- Sugar: 10g
- Protein: 9g
- Vitamin A: 450%
- Vitamin C: 90%
- Calcium: 8%
- Iron: 2mg

Blueberry Almond Butter Smoothie

Prep Time: 5 mins

Total Time: 5 mins

Servings: 1

Ingredients: 1 cup almond milk

- 1 frozen banana, ½ cup frozen blueberries
- 2 tablespoons almond butter
- 1 tablespoon honey or maple syrup

- Optional: 1 tablespoon chia seeds

Directions:

1. In a blender, combine almond milk, frozen banana, frozen blueberries, almond butter, honey or maple syrup, and optional chia seeds.
2. Blend until smooth and creamy.
3. Pour into a glass and serve immediately.

Nutrition Facts (per serving):

- Calories: 380
- Fat: 17g
- Saturated fat: 1.5g
- Cholesterol: 0mg
- Sodium: 170mg
- Carbohydrate: 53g
- Fiber: 9g
- Sugar: 33g
- Protein: 9g
- Calcium: 45%
- Iron: 1mg

Turkey Sausage and Veggie Breakfast Skillet

Prep Time: 10 mins

Total Time: 20 mins

Servings: 2

Ingredients: 4 turkey sausage links, sliced

- 1 bell pepper, diced, ½ onion, diced
- 2 cloves garlic, minced
- 2 cups baby spinach leaves

- 4 large eggs, 2 tablespoons olive oil
- Salt and pepper to taste

Directions:

1. Heat olive oil in a skillet over medium heat. Add the sliced turkey sausage and cook until browned.
2. Add the diced bell pepper, onion, and minced garlic to the skillet. Cook until the vegetables are softened.
3. Stir in the baby spinach leaves and cook until wilted.
4. Create four wells in the skillet and crack an egg into each well. Cook until the egg whites are set but the yolks are still runny.
5. Season with salt and pepper to taste.
6. Serve hot straight from the skillet.

Nutrition Facts (per serving):

- Calories: 320
- Fat: 22g
- Saturated fat: 5g
- Cholesterol: 380mg
- Sodium: 520mg
- Carbohydrate: 11g
- Fiber: 3g
- Sugar: 4g
- Protein: 21g
- Vitamin A: 100%
- Vitamin C: 70%
- Calcium: 10%
- Iron: 3mg

Coconut Mango Chia Pudding

Prep Time: 5 mins

Total Time: 4 hours 5 mins (overnight)

Servings: 2

Ingredients:

- ½ cup chia seeds
- 1½ cups coconut milk
- 1 ripe mango, diced
- 2 tablespoons shredded coconut
- 1 tablespoon honey or maple syrup

Directions:

1. In a bowl, combine chia seeds and coconut milk. Stir well to combine.
2. Cover and refrigerate for at least 4 hours or overnight, stirring occasionally, until thickened.
3. In serving glasses or bowls, layer the chia pudding with diced mango and shredded coconut.
4. Drizzle with honey or maple syrup before serving.

Nutrition Facts (per serving):

- Calories: 320
- Fat: 22g
- Saturated fat: 15g
- Cholesterol: 0mg
- Sodium: 20mg
- Carbohydrate: 32g
- Fiber: 12g
- Sugar: 16g

- Protein: 7g
- Calcium: 35%
- Iron: 3mg

Veggie and Feta Breakfast Wrap

Prep Time: 10 mins

Total Time: 15 mins

Servings: 1

Ingredients:

- 1 whole grain wrap
- 2 large eggs
- ½ cup diced bell peppers
- ½ cup diced onions
- ½ cup spinach leaves
- 2 tablespoons crumbled feta cheese
- 1 tablespoon olive oil
- Salt and pepper to taste

Directions:

1. In a skillet over medium heat, cook the eggs to your desired doneness (scrambled, fried, or poached).
2. Remove the eggs from the skillet and set aside.
3. In the same skillet, add the diced bell peppers, onions, and spinach leaves. Cook until the vegetables are softened.
4. Warm the whole grain wrap in the skillet or microwave.
5. Assemble the wrap by layering the cooked eggs, sautéed vegetables, and crumbled feta cheese in the center of the wrap.
6. Season with salt and pepper to taste.
7. Fold the sides of the wrap over the filling and roll up tightly.

8. Serve hot and enjoy!

Nutrition Facts (per serving):

- Calories: 380
- Fat: 20g
- Saturated fat: 6g
- Cholesterol: 380mg
- Sodium: 420mg
- Carbohydrate: 30g
- Fiber: 6g
- Sugar: 5g
- Protein: 18g
- Vitamin A: 80%
- Vitamin C: 150%
- Calcium: 20%
- Iron: 3mg

LUNCH RECIPES

Grilled Chicken Quinoa Salad

Prep Time: 15 mins

Total Time: 30 mins

Servings: 4

Ingredients:

- 1 cup quinoa
- 2 cups water or chicken broth
- 2 boneless, skinless chicken breasts
- 2 tablespoons olive oil
- 1 teaspoon garlic powder
- ½ teaspoon paprika
- Salt and pepper to taste
- 4 cups mixed salad greens
- 1 cup cherry tomatoes, halved
- 1 cucumber, diced
- ½ red onion, thinly sliced
- ¼ cup crumbled feta cheese
- Balsamic vinaigrette dressing

Directions:

1. Rinse quinoa under cold water and drain. In a saucepan, bring water or chicken broth to a boil. Add quinoa, reduce heat to low, cover, and simmer for 15 minutes or until quinoa is cooked and water is absorbed. Remove from heat and let it sit for 5 minutes before fluffing with a fork.

2. Preheat grill or grill pan over medium-high heat. Season chicken breasts with olive oil, garlic powder, paprika, salt, and

pepper. Grill chicken for 6-8 minutes per side or until cooked through. Let it rest for a few minutes before slicing.

3. In a large mixing bowl, combine cooked quinoa, mixed salad greens, cherry tomatoes, cucumber, red onion, and crumbled feta cheese. Toss with balsamic vinaigrette dressing.

4. Serve grilled chicken slices on top of the quinoa salad. Enjoy!

Nutrition Facts (per serving):

- Calories: 380
- Fat: 14g
- Saturated fat: 3g
- Cholesterol: 65mg
- Sodium: 250mg
- Carbohydrate: 35g
- Fiber: 6g
- Sugar: 4g
- Protein: 30g
- Vitamin A: 60%
- Vitamin C: 40%
- Calcium: 15%
- Iron: 3mg

Mediterranean Chickpea Salad

Prep Time: 15 mins

Total Time: 15 mins

Servings: 4

Ingredients:

- 2 cans (15 oz each) chickpeas, drained and rinsed
- 1 cup cherry tomatoes, halved

- 1 cucumber, diced
- ½ red onion, thinly sliced
- ½ cup Kalamata olives, pitted and sliced
- ¼ cup chopped fresh parsley
- 2 tablespoons extra virgin olive oil
- 1 tablespoon red wine vinegar
- 1 teaspoon dried oregano
- Salt and pepper to taste
- Crumbled feta cheese (optional)

Directions:

1. In a large mixing bowl, combine chickpeas, cherry tomatoes, cucumber, red onion, Kalamata olives, and chopped parsley.
2. Drizzle extra virgin olive oil and red wine vinegar over the salad. Sprinkle with dried oregano, salt, and pepper.
3. Toss until all ingredients are well combined and evenly coated with the dressing.
4. Top with crumbled feta cheese if desired.
5. Serve chilled or at room temperature.

Nutrition Facts (per serving):

- Calories: 280
- Fat: 10g
- Saturated fat: 1.5g
- Cholesterol: 0mg
- Sodium: 480mg
- Carbohydrate: 38g
- Fiber: 10g
- Sugar: 7g

- Protein: 10g
- Vitamin A: 15%
- Vitamin C: 25%
- Calcium: 10%
- Iron: 3mg

Teriyaki Tofu Stir-Fry

Prep Time: 15 mins

Total Time: 25 mins

Servings: 4

Ingredients:

- 1 block (14 oz) firm tofu, pressed and cubed
- 2 tablespoons low-sodium soy sauce
- 1 tablespoon honey or maple syrup
- 1 tablespoon rice vinegar
- 1 tablespoon sesame oil
- 1 teaspoon minced garlic
- 1 teaspoon minced ginger
- 2 tablespoons olive oil
- 2 cups mixed vegetables (broccoli florets, bell peppers, snap peas)
- Cooked brown rice or quinoa for serving
- Sesame seeds and sliced green onions for garnish

Directions:

1. In a bowl, whisk together low-sodium soy sauce, honey or maple syrup, rice vinegar, sesame oil, minced garlic, and minced ginger. Set aside.

2. Heat olive oil in a large skillet or wok over medium-high heat. Add cubed tofu and cook until golden brown on all sides.

3. Add mixed vegetables to the skillet and stir-fry until tender-crisp.

4. Pour the teriyaki sauce over the tofu and vegetables. Cook for another 2-3 minutes, stirring occasionally, until the sauce thickens and coats the tofu and vegetables.

5. Serve the teriyaki tofu stir-fry over cooked brown rice or quinoa. Garnish with sesame seeds and sliced green onions.

Nutrition Facts (per serving):

- Calories: 320
- Fat: 15g
- Saturated fat: 2g
- Cholesterol: 0mg
- Sodium: 430mg
- Carbohydrate: 28g
- Fiber: 6g
- Sugar: 9g
- Protein: 20g
- Vitamin A: 60%
- Vitamin C: 80%
- Calcium: 20%
- Iron: 3mg

Salmon and Avocado Salad

Prep Time: 10 mins

Total Time: 20 mins

Servings: 2

Ingredients: 2 salmon fillets (6 oz each)

- 2 cups mixed salad greens
- 1 avocado, sliced
- ½ cup cherry tomatoes, halved
- ¼ cup sliced red onion, 2 tablespoons chopped fresh dill
- 2 tablespoons extra virgin olive oil
- 1 tablespoon lemon juice
- Salt and pepper to taste

Directions:

1. Preheat oven to 400°F (200°C). Season salmon fillets with salt and pepper. Place on a baking sheet lined with parchment paper.
2. Bake salmon in the preheated oven for 12-15 minutes, or until cooked through and flakes easily with a fork.
3. In a large mixing bowl, combine mixed salad greens, sliced avocado, cherry tomatoes, sliced red onion, and chopped fresh dill.
4. In a small bowl, whisk together extra virgin olive oil and lemon juice to make the dressing. Season with salt and pepper.
5. Divide the salad mixture between two plates. Top each salad with a baked salmon fillet.
6. Drizzle the lemon vinaigrette over the salad and serve immediately.

Nutrition Facts (per serving):

- Calories: 420
- Fat: 28g
- Saturated fat: 4.5g

- Cholesterol: 90mg
- Sodium: 110mg
- Carbohydrate: 14g
- Fiber: 8g
- Sugar: 3g
- Protein: 34g
- Vitamin A: 90%
- Vitamin C: 35%
- Calcium: 6%
- Iron: 2mg

Veggie and Lentil Soup

Prep Time: 10 mins

Total Time: 40 mins

Servings: 4

Ingredients: 1 cup dried green lentils, rinsed and drained

- 4 cups vegetable broth
- 1 tablespoon olive oil
- 1 onion, diced
- 2 carrots, diced
- 2 celery stalks, diced
- 2 cloves garlic, minced
- 1 teaspoon ground cumin
- ½ teaspoon smoked paprika
- ½ teaspoon dried thyme
- Salt and pepper to taste
- Fresh parsley for garnish

Directions:

1. In a large pot, heat olive oil over medium heat. Add diced onion, carrots, and celery. Cook until softened, about 5 minutes.
2. Add minced garlic, ground cumin, smoked paprika, and dried thyme. Cook for another 1-2 minutes until fragrant.
3. Stir in dried green lentils and vegetable broth. Bring to a boil, then reduce heat to low, cover, and simmer for 25-30 minutes, or until lentils are tender.
4. Season with salt and pepper to taste.
5. Serve hot, garnished with fresh parsley.

Nutrition Facts (per serving):

- Calories: 250
- Fat: 4g
- Saturated fat: 0.5g
- Cholesterol: 0mg
- Sodium: 710mg
- Carbohydrate: 38g
- Fiber: 17g
- Sugar: 5g
- Protein: 14g
- Vitamin A: 120%
- Vitamin C: 15%
- Calcium: 6%
- Iron: 4mg

Turkey and Vegetable Wrap

Prep Time: 10 mins

Total Time: 15 mins

Servings: 2

Ingredients: 4 whole wheat or spinach tortillas

- 8 slices turkey breast
- ½ cup hummus
- 1 cup mixed salad greens
- 1 tomato, sliced
- ½ cucumber, thinly sliced
- ¼ red onion, thinly sliced
- ½ avocado, sliced
- Salt and pepper to taste

Directions:

1. Lay out the tortillas on a clean surface. Spread hummus evenly over each tortilla.
2. Divide the turkey slices evenly among the tortillas, placing them in the center.
3. Layer mixed salad greens, tomato slices, cucumber slices, red onion slices, and avocado slices over the turkey.
4. Season with salt and pepper to taste.
5. Roll up each tortilla tightly, folding in the sides as you go to create a wrap.
6. Slice each wrap in half diagonally and serve immediately.

Nutrition Facts (per serving):

- Calories: 320
- Fat: 14g

- Saturated fat: 2g
- Cholesterol: 35mg
- Sodium: 480mg
- Carbohydrate: 30g
- Fiber: 8g
- Sugar: 4g
- Protein: 20g
- Vitamin A: 60%
- Vitamin C: 25%
- Calcium: 10%
- Iron: 3mg

Quinoa Stuffed Bell Peppers

Prep Time: 15 mins

Total Time: 45 mins

Servings: 4

Ingredients:

- 4 bell peppers, any color
- 1 cup quinoa
- 2 cups water or vegetable broth
- 1 tablespoon olive oil
- 1 onion, diced
- 2 cloves garlic, minced
- 1 zucchini, diced
- 1 tomato, diced
- 1 cup cooked black beans
- 1 teaspoon chili powder
- ½ teaspoon ground cumin

- Salt and pepper to taste
- ½ cup shredded cheese (optional)

Directions:

1. Preheat oven to 375°F (190°C). Cut the tops off the bell peppers and remove the seeds and membranes.
2. In a saucepan, bring water or vegetable broth to a boil. Add quinoa, reduce heat to low, cover, and simmer for 15 minutes or until quinoa is cooked and water is absorbed.
3. Heat olive oil in a skillet over medium heat. Add diced onion and minced garlic, and sauté until translucent.
4. Add diced zucchini, tomato, cooked black beans, chili powder, ground cumin, salt, and pepper to the skillet. Cook for another 5 minutes until vegetables are tender.
5. Stir in cooked quinoa until well combined.
6. Stuff each bell pepper with the quinoa and vegetable mixture.
7. Place stuffed bell peppers in a baking dish. If using cheese, sprinkle shredded cheese over the tops of the peppers.
8. Bake in the preheated oven for 20-25 minutes, or until peppers are tender and cheese is melted and bubbly.
9. Serve hot.

Nutrition Facts (per serving):

- Calories: 280
- Fat: 7g
- Saturated fat: 2g
- Cholesterol: 5mg
- Sodium: 250mg
- Carbohydrate: 45g

- Fiber: 10g
- Sugar: 6g
- Protein: 12g
- Vitamin A: 120%
- Vitamin C: 220%
- Calcium: 10%
- Iron: 3mg

Veggie and Hummus Wrap

Prep Time: 10 mins

Total Time: 10 mins

Servings: 2

Ingredients: 2 large whole wheat or spinach tortillas

- ½ cup hummus, 1 cup mixed salad greens
- ½ cucumber, thinly sliced
- ½ bell pepper, thinly sliced
- ½ carrot, grated
- ¼ red onion, thinly sliced
- Salt and pepper to taste

Directions:

1. Lay out the tortillas on a clean surface. Spread hummus evenly over each tortilla.
2. Layer mixed salad greens, cucumber slices, bell pepper slices, grated carrot, and red onion slices over the hummus.
3. Season with salt and pepper to taste.
4. Roll up each tortilla tightly, folding in the sides as you go to create a wrap.
5. Slice each wrap in half diagonally and serve immediately.

Nutrition Facts (per serving):

- Calories: 260
- Fat: 10g
- Saturated fat: 1.5g
- Cholesterol: 0mg
- Sodium: 490mg
- Carbohydrate: 35g
- Fiber: 8g
- Sugar: 6g
- Protein: 10g
- Vitamin A: 90%
- Vitamin C: 70%
- Calcium: 8%
- Iron: 2mg

Mediterranean Chickpea Wrap

Prep Time: 10 mins

Total Time: 15 mins

Servings: 2

Ingredients: 2 large whole wheat or spinach tortillas

- 1 cup cooked chickpeas
- ½ cup hummus, ½ cup diced cucumber
- ½ cup diced tomato
- ¼ cup sliced Kalamata olives
- 2 tablespoons chopped fresh parsley
- 2 tablespoons crumbled feta cheese (optional)
- Salt and pepper to taste

Directions:

1. Lay out the tortillas on a clean surface. Spread hummus evenly over each tortilla.
2. Divide cooked chickpeas evenly between the tortillas, mashing slightly with a fork.
3. Top with diced cucumber, diced tomato, sliced Kalamata olives, chopped fresh parsley, and crumbled feta cheese if using.
4. Season with salt and pepper to taste.
5. Roll up each tortilla tightly, folding in the sides as you go to create a wrap.
6. Slice each wrap in half diagonally and serve immediately.

Nutrition Facts (per serving):

- Calories: 320
- Fat: 12g
- Saturated fat: 2g
- Cholesterol: 5mg
- Sodium: 480mg
- Carbohydrate: 40g
- Fiber: 10g
- Sugar: 6g
- Protein: 12g
- Vitamin A: 80%
- Vitamin C: 30%
- Calcium: 15%
- Iron: 3mg

Shrimp and Avocado Salad Wrap

Prep Time: 10 mins

Total Time: 15 mins

Servings: 2

Ingredients:

- 2 large whole wheat or spinach tortillas
- 8 oz cooked shrimp, peeled and deveined
- 1 avocado, sliced
- 1 cup mixed salad greens
- ½ cup diced tomato
- ¼ cup diced red onion
- 2 tablespoons chopped fresh cilantro
- 2 tablespoons Greek yogurt
- 1 tablespoon lime juice
- Salt and pepper to taste

Directions:

1. Lay out the tortillas on a clean surface.
2. In a small bowl, mash the avocado with Greek yogurt, lime juice, salt, and pepper to make the dressing.
3. Spread the avocado dressing evenly over each tortilla.
4. Divide cooked shrimp, mixed salad greens, diced tomato, diced red onion, and chopped fresh cilantro evenly between the tortillas.
5. Roll up each tortilla tightly, folding in the sides as you go to create a wrap.
6. Slice each wrap in half diagonally and serve immediately.

Nutrition Facts (per serving):

- Calories: 300
- Fat: 12g
- Saturated fat: 2g
- Cholesterol: 150mg
- Sodium: 390mg
- Carbohydrate: 30g
- Fiber: 8g
- Sugar: 5g
- Protein: 20g
- Vitamin A: 70%
- Vitamin C: 45%
- Calcium: 10%
- Iron: 3mg

Greek Chicken Salad Bowl

Prep Time: 15 mins

Total Time: 30 mins

Servings: 2

Ingredients:

- 2 boneless, skinless chicken breasts
- 2 tablespoons olive oil
- 1 teaspoon dried oregano
- Salt and pepper to taste
- 2 cups mixed salad greens
- ½ cucumber, diced
- ½ cup cherry tomatoes, halved
- ¼ cup sliced red onion

- ½ cup cooked quinoa
- ¼ cup crumbled feta cheese
- 2 tablespoons Kalamata olives, sliced
- 2 tablespoons Greek yogurt
- 1 tablespoon lemon juice
- 1 tablespoon chopped fresh dill

Directions:

1. Preheat oven to 400°F (200°C). Place chicken breasts on a baking sheet lined with parchment paper. Drizzle with olive oil and sprinkle with dried oregano, salt, and pepper.
2. Bake chicken in the preheated oven for 20-25 minutes, or until cooked through and no longer pink in the center. Let cool slightly, then slice into strips.
3. In a large mixing bowl, combine mixed salad greens, diced cucumber, cherry tomatoes, sliced red onion, cooked quinoa, crumbled feta cheese, and sliced Kalamata olives.
4. In a small bowl, whisk together Greek yogurt, lemon juice, and chopped fresh dill to make the dressing.
5. Divide the salad mixture between two bowls. Top each bowl with sliced chicken breast and drizzle with the Greek yogurt dressing.
6. Serve immediately.

Nutrition Facts (per serving):

- Calories: 380
- Fat: 18g
- Saturated fat: 5g
- Cholesterol: 90mg

- Sodium: 450mg

- Carbohydrate: 20g

- Fiber: 4g

- Sugar: 4g

- Protein: 34g

- Vitamin A: 70%

- Vitamin C: 30%

- Calcium: 15%

- Iron: 3mg

Tuna and White Bean Salad

Prep Time: 10 mins

Total Time: 15 mins

Servings: 2

Ingredients: 1 can (5 oz) tuna in water, drained

- 1 can (15 oz) cannellini beans, drained and rinsed

- ½ cup diced red bell pepper

- ½ cup diced celery, ¼ cup chopped fresh parsley

- 2 tablespoons extra virgin olive oil

- 1 tablespoon red wine vinegar

- 1 teaspoon Dijon mustard

- Salt and pepper to taste

- Mixed salad greens for serving

Directions:

1. In a large mixing bowl, combine drained tuna, cannellini beans, diced red bell pepper, diced celery, and chopped fresh parsley.

2. In a small bowl, whisk together extra virgin olive oil, red wine vinegar, Dijon mustard, salt, and pepper to make the dressing.

3. Pour the dressing over the tuna and white bean mixture. Toss gently to coat.

4. Serve the tuna and white bean salad over a bed of mixed salad greens.

Nutrition Facts (per serving):

- Calories: 320
- Fat: 14g
- Saturated fat: 2g
- Cholesterol: 25mg
- Sodium: 460mg
- Carbohydrate: 30g
- Fiber: 10g
- Sugar: 1g
- Protein: 22g
- Vitamin A: 45%
- Vitamin C: 90%
- Calcium: 15%
- Iron: 4mg

Grilled Vegetable Quinoa Bowl

Prep Time: 15 mins

Total Time: 30 mins

Servings: 2

Ingredients: 1 cup quinoa, rinsed and drained

- 2 cups water or vegetable broth
- 1 medium zucchini, sliced

- 1 medium yellow squash, sliced
- 1 red bell pepper, sliced
- 1 yellow bell pepper, sliced
- 1 red onion, sliced
- 2 tablespoons olive oil
- 2 tablespoons balsamic vinegar
- Salt and pepper to taste
- ¼ cup crumbled feta cheese
- 2 tablespoons chopped fresh basil

Directions:

1. In a saucepan, bring water or vegetable broth to a boil. Add quinoa, reduce heat to low, cover, and simmer for 15 minutes or until quinoa is cooked and water is absorbed.
2. Preheat grill or grill pan to medium-high heat.
3. In a large mixing bowl, toss sliced zucchini, yellow squash, red bell pepper, yellow bell pepper, and red onion with olive oil, balsamic vinegar, salt, and pepper.
4. Grill the vegetables for 5-7 minutes per side, or until tender and charred.
5. Divide cooked quinoa between two bowls. Top each bowl with grilled vegetables, crumbled feta cheese, and chopped fresh basil.
6. Serve immediately.

Nutrition Facts (per serving):

- Calories: 380
- Fat: 14g
- Saturated fat: 4g

- Cholesterol: 15mg
- Sodium: 380mg
- Carbohydrate: 52g
- Fiber: 9g
- Sugar: 9g
- Protein: 12g
- Vitamin A: 70%
- Vitamin C: 260%
- Calcium: 15%
- Iron: 4mg

Chicken and Quinoa Salad

Prep Time: 15 mins

Total Time: 30 mins

Servings: 2

Ingredients:

- 2 boneless, skinless chicken breasts
- 1 tablespoon olive oil
- Salt and pepper to taste
- 1 cup cooked quinoa
- 2 cups mixed salad greens
- ½ cucumber, sliced
- ½ cup cherry tomatoes, halved
- ¼ cup sliced red onion
- 2 tablespoons chopped fresh parsley
- 2 tablespoons extra virgin olive oil
- 1 tablespoon lemon juice
- 1 clove garlic, minced

- ½ teaspoon dried oregano

Directions:

1. Preheat oven to 400°F (200°C). Place chicken breasts on a baking sheet lined with parchment paper. Drizzle with olive oil and season with salt, pepper, and dried oregano.

2. Bake chicken in the preheated oven for 20-25 minutes, or until cooked through and no longer pink in the center. Let cool slightly, then slice into strips.

3. In a large mixing bowl, combine cooked quinoa, mixed salad greens, sliced cucumber, cherry tomatoes, sliced red onion, and chopped fresh parsley.

4. In a small bowl, whisk together extra virgin olive oil, lemon juice, minced garlic, salt, and pepper to make the dressing.

5. Divide the salad mixture between two plates. Top each salad with sliced chicken breast and drizzle with the lemon garlic dressing.

6. Serve immediately.

Nutrition Facts (per serving):

- Calories: 350
- Fat: 15g
- Saturated fat: 2.5g
- Cholesterol: 90mg
- Sodium: 160mg
- Carbohydrate: 25g
- Fiber: 4g
- Sugar: 4g
- Protein: 30g

- Vitamin A: 60%
- Vitamin C: 40%
- Calcium: 8%
- Iron: 3mg

Mediterranean Chickpea Salad

Prep Time: 15 mins

Total Time: 15 mins

Servings: 2

Ingredients:

- 1 can (15 oz) chickpeas, drained and rinsed
- ½ English cucumber, diced
- ½ cup cherry tomatoes, halved
- ¼ cup diced red onion
- ¼ cup sliced Kalamata olives
- 2 tablespoons chopped fresh parsley
- 2 tablespoons extra virgin olive oil
- 1 tablespoon red wine vinegar
- 1 teaspoon dried oregano
- Salt and pepper to taste
- 2 cups mixed salad greens

Directions:

1. In a large mixing bowl, combine drained chickpeas, diced cucumber, cherry tomatoes, diced red onion, sliced Kalamata olives, and chopped fresh parsley.

2. In a small bowl, whisk together extra virgin olive oil, red wine vinegar, dried oregano, salt, and pepper to make the dressing.

3. Pour the dressing over the chickpea mixture. Toss gently to coat.

4. Serve the chickpea salad over a bed of mixed salad greens.

Nutrition Facts (per serving):

- Calories: 280
- Fat: 15g
- Saturated fat: 2g
- Cholesterol: 0mg
- Sodium: 420mg
- Carbohydrate: 30g
- Fiber: 8g
- Sugar: 6g
- Protein: 8g
- Vitamin A: 45%
- Vitamin C: 30%
- Calcium: 8%
- Iron: 2mg

DINNER RECIPES

Lemon Herb Grilled Salmon

Prep Time: 10 mins

Total Time: 20 mins

Servings: 2

Ingredients:

- 2 salmon fillets
- 2 tablespoons olive oil
- 1 lemon, juiced and zested
- 2 cloves garlic, minced
- 1 tablespoon chopped fresh parsley
- 1 tablespoon chopped fresh dill
- Salt and pepper to taste

Directions:

1. Preheat grill to medium-high heat.
2. In a small bowl, whisk together olive oil, lemon juice, lemon zest, minced garlic, chopped parsley, chopped dill, salt, and pepper.
3. Place salmon fillets on a piece of aluminum foil. Brush the lemon herb mixture over the salmon.
4. Grill salmon for 4-5 minutes per side, or until fish flakes easily with a fork.
5. Serve grilled salmon with your choice of side dishes.

Nutrition Facts (per serving):

- Calories: 320
- Fat: 20g
- Saturated fat: 3.5g

- Cholesterol: 90mg

- Sodium: 80mg

- Carbohydrate: 2g

- Fiber: 0.5g

- Sugar: 0.5g

- Protein: 30g

- Vitamin A: 10%

- Vitamin C: 25%

- Calcium: 4%

- Iron: 1mg

Turkey and Quinoa Stuffed Bell Peppers

Prep Time: 15 mins

Total Time: 45 mins

Servings: 4

Ingredients:

- 4 bell peppers (any color), halved and seeds removed

- 1 cup cooked quinoa

- 1 lb ground turkey

- 1 small onion, diced

- 2 cloves garlic, minced

- 1 teaspoon dried oregano

- 1 teaspoon ground cumin

- Salt and pepper to taste

- 1 cup tomato sauce

- ½ cup shredded mozzarella cheese

- Fresh parsley for garnish

Directions:

1. Preheat oven to 375°F (190°C).

2. In a large skillet, cook ground turkey over medium heat until browned. Add diced onion, minced garlic, dried oregano, ground cumin, salt, and pepper. Cook until onion is softened.

3. Stir in cooked quinoa and tomato sauce. Cook for another 2-3 minutes.

4. Arrange bell pepper halves in a baking dish. Spoon the turkey and quinoa mixture into each pepper half.

5. Cover the baking dish with aluminum foil and bake in the preheated oven for 25-30 minutes.

6. Remove foil, sprinkle shredded mozzarella cheese over the stuffed peppers, and bake for an additional 5 minutes, or until cheese is melted and bubbly.

7. Garnish with fresh parsley before serving.

Nutrition Facts (per serving):

- Calories: 320
- Fat: 12g
- Saturated fat: 4g
- Cholesterol: 80mg
- Sodium: 320mg
- Carbohydrate: 20g
- Fiber: 4g
- Sugar: 5g
- Protein: 30g
- Vitamin A: 70%
- Vitamin C: 190%

- Calcium: 15%
- Iron: 3mg

Baked Lemon Garlic Chicken

Prep Time: 10 mins

Total Time: 35 mins

Servings: 2

Ingredients:

- 2 boneless, skinless chicken breasts
- 2 tablespoons olive oil
- 2 tablespoons lemon juice
- 2 cloves garlic, minced
- 1 teaspoon dried oregano
- Salt and pepper to taste
- Lemon slices for garnish
- Fresh parsley for garnish

Directions:

1. Preheat oven to 400°F (200°C).
2. In a small bowl, whisk together olive oil, lemon juice, minced garlic, dried oregano, salt, and pepper.
3. Place chicken breasts in a baking dish. Pour the lemon garlic mixture over the chicken.
4. Bake in the preheated oven for 25-30 minutes, or until chicken is cooked through and juices run clear.
5. Garnish with lemon slices and fresh parsley before serving.

Nutrition Facts (per serving):

- Calories: 280
- Fat: 14g

- Saturated fat: 2.5g
- Cholesterol: 90mg
- Sodium: 120mg
- Carbohydrate: 2g
- Fiber: 0.5g
- Sugar: 0.5g
- Protein: 35g
- Vitamin A: 4%
- Vitamin C: 15%
- Calcium: 2%
- Iron: 2mg

Vegetarian Stir-Fry

Prep Time: 15 mins

Total Time: 25 mins

Servings: 4

Ingredients:

- 2 tablespoons sesame oil
- 2 cups mixed vegetables (bell peppers, broccoli, snap peas, carrots, etc.), sliced
- 1 cup sliced mushrooms
- 1 cup sliced tofu
- 2 cloves garlic, minced
- 1 tablespoon grated ginger
- 3 tablespoons soy sauce
- 1 tablespoon rice vinegar
- 1 tablespoon honey or maple syrup
- Cooked brown rice for serving

- Sesame seeds for garnish
- Sliced green onions for garnish

Directions:

1. Heat sesame oil in a large skillet or wok over medium-high heat.
2. Add mixed vegetables, sliced mushrooms, and sliced tofu to the skillet. Cook, stirring frequently, for 5-7 minutes, or until vegetables are tender-crisp.
3. Add minced garlic and grated ginger to the skillet. Cook for another 1-2 minutes.
4. In a small bowl, whisk together soy sauce, rice vinegar, and honey or maple syrup. Pour the sauce over the vegetables and tofu in the skillet. Stir to coat evenly.
5. Serve vegetarian stir-fry over cooked brown rice. Garnish with sesame seeds and sliced green onions.

Nutrition Facts (per serving):

- Calories: 250
- Fat: 12g
- Saturated fat: 2g
- Cholesterol: 0mg
- Sodium: 450mg
- Carbohydrate: 28g
- Fiber: 6g
- Sugar: 10g
- Protein: 12g
- Vitamin A: 60%
- Vitamin C: 80%

- Calcium: 10%
- Iron: 2mg

Shrimp and Asparagus Stir-Fry

Prep Time: 15 mins

Total Time: 25 mins

Servings: 2

Ingredients:

- 1 tablespoon sesame oil
- 1 lb large shrimp, peeled and deveined
- 1 bunch asparagus, trimmed and cut into 2-inch pieces
- 2 cloves garlic, minced
- 1 tablespoon grated ginger
- 2 tablespoons soy sauce
- 1 tablespoon oyster sauce
- 1 teaspoon cornstarch
- Cooked brown rice for serving
- Sliced green onions for garnish
- Sesame seeds for garnish

Directions:

1. Heat sesame oil in a large skillet or wok over medium-high heat.
2. Add shrimp to the skillet and cook for 2-3 minutes per side, until pink and cooked through. Remove shrimp from skillet and set aside.
3. In the same skillet, add asparagus pieces and cook for 3-4 minutes, or until crisp-tender.

4. Add minced garlic and grated ginger to the skillet. Cook for another 1-2 minutes.

5. In a small bowl, whisk together soy sauce, oyster sauce, and cornstarch. Pour the sauce over the asparagus in the skillet.

6. Return cooked shrimp to the skillet and stir to coat everything evenly with the sauce.

7. Serve shrimp and asparagus stir-fry over cooked brown rice. Garnish with sliced green onions and sesame seeds.

Nutrition Facts (per serving):

- Calories: 280
- Fat: 10g
- Saturated fat: 2g
- Cholesterol: 180mg
- Sodium: 700mg
- Carbohydrate: 16g
- Fiber: 5g
- Sugar: 5g
- Protein: 30g
- Vitamin A: 30%
- Vitamin C: 50%
- Calcium: 15%
- Iron: 3mg

Balsamic Glazed Chicken with Roasted Vegetables

Prep Time: 15 mins

Total Time: 45 mins

Servings: 2

Ingredients:

- 2 boneless, skinless chicken breasts
- 2 tablespoons balsamic vinegar
- 1 tablespoon olive oil
- 2 cloves garlic, minced
- 1 teaspoon dried thyme
- Salt and pepper to taste
- 1 cup cherry tomatoes, halved
- 1 bell pepper, sliced
- 1 zucchini, sliced
- 1 tablespoon chopped fresh basil
- 1 tablespoon grated Parmesan cheese (optional)

Directions:

1. Preheat oven to 400°F (200°C).
2. In a small bowl, whisk together balsamic vinegar, olive oil, minced garlic, dried thyme, salt, and pepper.
3. Place chicken breasts in a baking dish. Brush the balsamic glaze over the chicken.
4. Arrange cherry tomatoes, sliced bell pepper, and sliced zucchini around the chicken in the baking dish. Drizzle with any remaining balsamic glaze.
5. Bake in the preheated oven for 25-30 minutes, or until chicken is cooked through and vegetables are tender.
6. Garnish with chopped fresh basil and grated Parmesan cheese before serving.

Nutrition Facts (per serving):

- Calories: 280
- Fat: 9g

- Saturated fat: 2g
- Cholesterol: 80mg
- Sodium: 220mg
- Carbohydrate: 10g
- Fiber: 3g
- Sugar: 6g
- Protein: 35g
- Vitamin A: 40%
- Vitamin C: 150%
- Calcium: 8%
- Iron: 2mg

Quinoa and Black Bean Stuffed Sweet Potatoes

Prep Time: 10 mins

Total Time: 50 mins

Servings: 2

Ingredients:

- 2 medium sweet potatoes
- 1 cup cooked quinoa
- ½ cup canned black beans, rinsed and drained
- ½ cup corn kernels
- ¼ cup diced red onion
- 1 teaspoon ground cumin
- 1 teaspoon chili powder
- Salt and pepper to taste
- ¼ cup chopped fresh cilantro
- 2 tablespoons Greek yogurt (optional)
- Lime wedges for serving

Directions:

1. Preheat oven to 400°F (200°C).

2. Scrub sweet potatoes and pierce with a fork. Place on a baking sheet and bake for 45-50 minutes, or until tender.

3. In a medium bowl, combine cooked quinoa, black beans, corn kernels, diced red onion, ground cumin, chili powder, salt, and pepper.

4. Once sweet potatoes are cooked, slice them open lengthwise and fluff the flesh with a fork.

5. Stuff each sweet potato with the quinoa and black bean mixture.

6. Garnish with chopped fresh cilantro and a dollop of Greek yogurt, if desired. Serve with lime wedges on the side.

Nutrition Facts (per serving):

- Calories: 320
- Fat: 2g
- Saturated fat: 0.5g
- Cholesterol: 0mg
- Sodium: 240mg
- Carbohydrate: 65g
- Fiber: 10g
- Sugar: 12g
- Protein: 10g
- Vitamin A: 750%
- Vitamin C: 25%
- Calcium: 10%
- Iron: 4mg

Grilled Vegetable Quesadillas

Prep Time: 15 mins

Total Time: 25 mins

Servings: 2

Ingredients:

- 4 whole wheat tortillas
- 1 cup shredded Monterey Jack cheese
- 1 zucchini, sliced
- 1 yellow squash, sliced
- 1 bell pepper, sliced
- 1 red onion, sliced
- 2 tablespoons olive oil
- Salt and pepper to taste
- Salsa, guacamole, and Greek yogurt for serving

Directions:

1. Preheat grill or grill pan over medium heat.
2. Brush zucchini, yellow squash, bell pepper, and red onion slices with olive oil. Season with salt and pepper.
3. Grill vegetables for 3-4 minutes per side, or until tender and lightly charred. Remove from grill and set aside.
4. Place one whole wheat tortilla on a flat surface. Sprinkle shredded Monterey Jack cheese evenly over the tortilla.
5. Arrange grilled vegetables over the cheese. Top with another tortilla.
6. Repeat with remaining tortillas and vegetables.
7. Grill quesadillas for 2-3 minutes per side, or until cheese is melted and tortillas are crispy.

8. Cut quesadillas into wedges and serve with salsa, guacamole, and Greek yogurt.

Nutrition Facts (per serving):

- Calories: 350
- Fat: 15g
- Saturated fat: 4.5g
- Cholesterol: 20mg
- Sodium: 500mg
- Carbohydrate: 45g
- Fiber: 8g
- Sugar: 6g
- Protein: 12g
- Vitamin A: 60%
- Vitamin C: 150%
- Calcium: 25%
- Iron: 3mg

Lentil and Vegetable Curry

Prep Time: 15 mins

Total Time: 40 mins

Servings: 4

Ingredients:

- 1 cup dry lentils, rinsed and drained
- 1 tablespoon olive oil
- 1 onion, diced
- 2 cloves garlic, minced
- 1 tablespoon grated ginger
- 1 tablespoon curry powder

- 1 teaspoon ground turmeric
- 1 teaspoon ground cumin
- 1 teaspoon ground coriander
- 1 can (14 oz) diced tomatoes
- 1 can (14 oz) coconut milk
- 2 cups mixed vegetables (bell peppers, carrots, peas, etc.)
- Salt and pepper to taste
- Cooked brown rice for serving
- Chopped fresh cilantro for garnish

Directions:

1. In a large pot, heat olive oil over medium heat. Add diced onion and cook until translucent.
2. Add minced garlic and grated ginger to the pot. Cook for another minute, until fragrant.
3. Stir in curry powder, ground turmeric, ground cumin, and ground coriander. Cook for 1-2 minutes, stirring constantly.
4. Add diced tomatoes (with their juices), coconut milk, and rinsed lentils to the pot. Bring to a simmer and cook for 20-25 minutes, or until lentils are tender.
5. Stir in mixed vegetables and cook for an additional 5-7 minutes, until vegetables are cooked through.
6. Season with salt and pepper to taste.
7. Serve lentil and vegetable curry over cooked brown rice. Garnish with chopped fresh cilantro.

Nutrition Facts (per serving):

- Calories: 380
- Fat: 18g

- Saturated fat: 12g
- Cholesterol: 0mg
- Sodium: 360mg
- Carbohydrate: 45g
- Fiber: 12g
- Sugar: 7g
- Protein: 15g
- Vitamin A: 70%
- Vitamin C: 40%
- Calcium: 10%
- Iron: 6mg

Salmon and Asparagus Foil Packets

Prep Time: 10 mins

Total Time: 25 mins

Servings: 2

Ingredients:

- 2 salmon fillets
- 1 bunch asparagus, trimmed
- 2 tablespoons olive oil
- 2 cloves garlic, minced
- 1 lemon, thinly sliced
- Salt and pepper to taste
- Chopped fresh parsley for garnish

Directions:

1. Preheat oven to 400°F (200°C).
2. Cut two large pieces of aluminum foil. Place one salmon fillet in the center of each piece of foil.

3. Arrange trimmed asparagus around the salmon fillets.

4. Drizzle olive oil over the salmon and asparagus. Sprinkle minced garlic over the top.

5. Season with salt and pepper to taste. Place lemon slices on top of the salmon.

6. Fold the foil over the salmon and asparagus to create packets, sealing the edges tightly.

7. Place foil packets on a baking sheet and bake in the preheated oven for 15-20 minutes, or until salmon is cooked through and asparagus is tender.

8. Carefully open the foil packets and transfer salmon and asparagus to serving plates. Garnish with chopped fresh parsley before serving.

Nutrition Facts (per serving):

- Calories: 320
- Fat: 20g
- Saturated fat: 3.5g
- Cholesterol: 80mg
- Sodium: 120mg
- Carbohydrate: 8g
- Fiber: 4g
- Sugar: 3g
- Protein: 30g
- Vitamin A: 20%
- Vitamin C: 60%
- Calcium: 8%
- Iron: 2mg

Turkey and Vegetable Stir-Fry

Prep Time: 15 mins

Total Time: 25 mins

Servings: 4

Ingredients:

- 1 lb lean ground turkey
- 1 tablespoon olive oil
- 2 cups broccoli florets
- 1 red bell pepper, sliced
- 1 yellow bell pepper, sliced
- 1 cup snap peas
- 2 cloves garlic, minced
- 2 tablespoons low-sodium soy sauce
- 1 tablespoon honey
- 1 teaspoon sesame oil
- Cooked quinoa or brown rice for serving

Directions:

1. Heat olive oil in a large skillet over medium-high heat. Add ground turkey and cook until browned and cooked through, breaking it apart with a spoon.

2. Add broccoli florets, sliced red bell pepper, sliced yellow bell pepper, snap peas, and minced garlic to the skillet. Cook for 5-7 minutes, or until vegetables are tender-crisp.

3. In a small bowl, whisk together low-sodium soy sauce, honey, and sesame oil. Pour the sauce over the turkey and vegetables in the skillet.

4. Stir everything together until well coated in the sauce.

5. Serve turkey and vegetable stir-fry over cooked quinoa or brown rice.

Nutrition Facts (per serving):

- Calories: 280
- Fat: 10g
- Saturated fat: 2g
- Cholesterol: 60mg
- Sodium: 350mg
- Carbohydrate: 20g
- Fiber: 5g
- Sugar: 8g
- Protein: 25g
- Vitamin A: 90%
- Vitamin C: 160%
- Calcium: 8%
- Iron: 3mg

Mediterranean Chickpea Salad

Prep Time: 10 mins

Total Time: 10 mins

Servings: 4

Ingredients:

- 1 can (15 oz) chickpeas, rinsed and drained
- 1 cucumber, diced
- 1 cup cherry tomatoes, halved
- ½ red onion, thinly sliced
- ¼ cup chopped fresh parsley
- ¼ cup chopped fresh mint

- 2 tablespoons extra virgin olive oil
- 1 tablespoon red wine vinegar
- 1 clove garlic, minced
- Salt and pepper to taste
- Crumbled feta cheese for serving (optional)
- Kalamata olives for serving (optional)

Directions:

1. In a large bowl, combine chickpeas, diced cucumber, halved cherry tomatoes, thinly sliced red onion, chopped fresh parsley, and chopped fresh mint.
2. In a small bowl, whisk together extra virgin olive oil, red wine vinegar, minced garlic, salt, and pepper.
3. Pour the dressing over the chickpea salad and toss to coat everything evenly.
4. Serve Mediterranean chickpea salad topped with crumbled feta cheese and Kalamata olives, if desired.

Nutrition Facts (per serving):

- Calories: 210
- Fat: 10g
- Saturated fat: 1.5g
- Cholesterol: 0mg
- Sodium: 350mg
- Carbohydrate: 24g
- Fiber: 6g
- Sugar: 5g
- Protein: 7g
- Vitamin A: 15%

- Vitamin C: 35%
- Calcium: 6%
- Iron: 2mg

Lemon Garlic Shrimp with Zucchini Noodles

Prep Time: 10 mins

Total Time: 20 mins

Servings: 2

Ingredients:

- 8 oz large shrimp, peeled and deveined
- 2 medium zucchini, spiralized into noodles
- 2 tablespoons olive oil
- 3 cloves garlic, minced
- Zest and juice of 1 lemon
- Salt and pepper to taste
- Chopped fresh parsley for garnish

Directions:

1. Heat olive oil in a large skillet over medium heat. Add minced garlic and cook for 1-2 minutes, until fragrant.
2. Add shrimp to the skillet and cook for 2-3 minutes per side, until pink and cooked through.
3. Add spiralized zucchini noodles to the skillet. Cook for 2-3 minutes, tossing frequently, until noodles are heated through and tender.
4. Stir in lemon zest and lemon juice. Season with salt and pepper to taste.
5. Serve lemon garlic shrimp over zucchini noodles, garnished with chopped fresh parsley.

Nutrition Facts (per serving):

- Calories: 250
- Fat: 14g
- Saturated fat: 2g
- Cholesterol: 180mg
- Sodium: 250mg
- Carbohydrate: 10g
- Fiber: 3g
- Sugar: 6g
- Protein: 25g
- Vitamin A: 20%
- Vitamin C: 50%
- Calcium: 10%
- Iron: 3mg

Stuffed Bell Peppers with Turkey and Quinoa

Prep Time: 15 mins

Total Time: 45 mins

Servings: 4

Ingredients:

- 4 large bell peppers
- 1 cup cooked quinoa
- 1 lb lean ground turkey
- 1 tablespoon olive oil
- 1 onion, diced
- 2 cloves garlic, minced
- 1 teaspoon dried oregano
- 1 teaspoon ground cumin

- ½ teaspoon paprika

- Salt and pepper to taste

- 1 cup tomato sauce

- ½ cup shredded mozzarella cheese

- Chopped fresh parsley for garnish

Directions:

1. Preheat oven to 375°F (190°C).

2. Cut the tops off the bell peppers and remove the seeds and membranes. Place the bell peppers in a baking dish.

3. In a large skillet, heat olive oil over medium heat. Add diced onion and cook until softened, about 5 minutes. Add minced garlic and cook for an additional minute.

4. Add ground turkey to the skillet and cook until browned, breaking it apart with a spoon.

5. Stir in cooked quinoa, dried oregano, ground cumin, paprika, salt, and pepper. Cook for 2-3 minutes.

6. Spoon the turkey and quinoa mixture into the bell peppers, dividing it evenly among them.

7. Pour tomato sauce over the stuffed bell peppers.

8. Cover the baking dish with foil and bake in the preheated oven for 30 minutes.

9. Remove foil and sprinkle shredded mozzarella cheese over the top of each stuffed bell pepper. Return to the oven and bake for an additional 10 minutes, or until cheese is melted and bubbly.

10. Garnish stuffed bell peppers with chopped fresh parsley before serving.

Nutrition Facts (per serving):

- Calories: 320
- Fat: 12g
- Saturated fat: 3.5g
- Cholesterol: 80mg
- Sodium: 450mg
- Carbohydrate: 30g
- Fiber: 7g
- Sugar: 8g
- Protein: 25g
- Vitamin A: 120%
- Vitamin C: 240%
- Calcium: 15%
- Iron: 4mg

Grilled Lemon Herb Chicken with Roasted Vegetables

Prep Time: 15 mins

Total Time: 35 mins

Servings: 4

Ingredients:

- 4 boneless, skinless chicken breasts
- 2 tablespoons olive oil
- 2 cloves garlic, minced
- Zest and juice of 1 lemon
- 1 teaspoon dried thyme
- 1 teaspoon dried rosemary
- 1 teaspoon dried oregano
- Salt and pepper to taste

- 2 cups mixed vegetables (such as bell peppers, zucchini, and cherry tomatoes), diced
- Cooking spray

Directions:

1. Preheat grill to medium-high heat.
2. In a small bowl, whisk together olive oil, minced garlic, lemon zest, lemon juice, dried thyme, dried rosemary, dried oregano, salt, and pepper.
3. Place chicken breasts in a shallow dish and pour the marinade over them, turning to coat evenly. Let marinate for 10-15 minutes.
4. Thread diced mixed vegetables onto skewers. Lightly coat with cooking spray.
5. Grill chicken breasts for 6-8 minutes per side, or until cooked through and no longer pink in the center.
6. During the last 5 minutes of grilling, add vegetable skewers to the grill and cook until vegetables are tender and lightly charred.
7. Remove chicken breasts and vegetable skewers from the grill and serve immediately.

Nutrition Facts (per serving):

- Calories: 280
- Fat: 12g
- Saturated fat: 2g
- Cholesterol: 80mg
- Sodium: 200mg
- Carbohydrate: 10g

- Fiber: 3g

- Sugar: 5g

- Protein: 30g

- Vitamin A: 80%

- Vitamin C: 100%

- Calcium: 6%

- Iron: 2mg

SNACKS AND DESSERTS RECIPES

Greek Yogurt Parfait

Prep Time: 5 mins

Total Time: 5 mins

Servings: 1

Ingredients:

- 1/2 cup plain Greek yogurt
- 1/4 cup mixed berries (such as strawberries, blueberries, and raspberries)
- 1 tablespoon honey or maple syrup
- 2 tablespoons granola
- Fresh mint leaves for garnish (optional)

Directions:

1. In a glass or bowl, layer Greek yogurt, mixed berries, and granola.
2. Drizzle honey or maple syrup over the top.
3. Garnish with fresh mint leaves if desired.
4. Serve immediately.

Nutrition Facts (per serving):

- Calories: 200
- Fat: 3g
- Saturated fat: 0g
- Cholesterol: 10mg
- Sodium: 40mg
- Carbohydrate: 30g
- Fiber: 3g
- Sugar: 20g

- Protein: 15g
- Vitamin C: 20%
- Calcium: 15%
- Iron: 2%

Avocado Chocolate Mousse

Prep Time: 10 mins

Total Time: 10 mins

Servings: 2

Ingredients:

- 1 ripe avocado, peeled and pitted
- 2 tablespoons unsweetened cocoa powder
- 2 tablespoons honey or maple syrup
- 1/2 teaspoon vanilla extract
- Pinch of salt
- Fresh berries for serving (optional)
- Shredded coconut for serving (optional)

Directions:

1. In a blender or food processor, combine ripe avocado, unsweetened cocoa powder, honey or maple syrup, vanilla extract, and a pinch of salt.
2. Blend until smooth and creamy, scraping down the sides as needed.
3. Divide the avocado chocolate mousse between two serving dishes.
4. Serve topped with fresh berries and shredded coconut if desired.
5. Refrigerate any leftovers for up to 2 days.

Nutrition Facts (per serving):

- Calories: 200
- Fat: 12g
- Saturated fat: 2g
- Cholesterol: 0mg
- Sodium: 5mg
- Carbohydrate: 25g
- Fiber: 7g
- Sugar: 15g
- Protein: 3g
- Vitamin C: 10%
- Calcium: 2%
- Iron: 2mg

Almond Butter Banana Bites

Prep Time: 5 mins

Total Time: 5 mins

Servings: 2

Ingredients: 1 large banana, peeled and sliced

- 2 tablespoons almond butter
- 2 teaspoons honey or maple syrup
- 1 tablespoon chopped almonds
- Pinch of cinnamon

Directions:

1. Spread almond butter on each banana slice.
2. Drizzle honey or maple syrup over the almond butter.
3. Sprinkle chopped almonds and a pinch of cinnamon on top.
4. Serve immediately as a snack or dessert.

Nutrition Facts (per serving):

- Calories: 150
- Fat: 8g
- Saturated fat: 1g
- Cholesterol: 0mg
- Sodium: 0mg
- Carbohydrate: 20g
- Fiber: 3g
- Sugar: 12g
- Protein: 3g
- Vitamin C: 8%
- Calcium: 4%
- Iron: 1mg

Berry Frozen Yogurt Bark

Prep Time: 10 mins

Total Time: 2 hrs 10 mins

Servings: 6

Ingredients: 2 cups plain Greek yogurt

- 2 tablespoons honey or maple syrup
- 1 cup mixed berries (such as strawberries, blueberries, and raspberries)
- 2 tablespoons shredded coconut
- 2 tablespoons chopped nuts (such as almonds or walnuts)

Directions:

1. In a bowl, mix together plain Greek yogurt and honey or maple syrup until well combined.
2. Line a baking sheet with parchment paper.

3. Spread the yogurt mixture evenly onto the parchment paper, about 1/4 inch thick.

4. Sprinkle mixed berries, shredded coconut, and chopped nuts over the yogurt mixture.

5. Place the baking sheet in the freezer and freeze for at least 2 hours, or until the yogurt bark is firm.

6. Once frozen, break the yogurt bark into pieces.

7. Serve immediately as a refreshing snack or dessert.

Nutrition Facts (per serving):

- Calories: 100
- Fat: 5g
- Saturated fat: 2g
- Cholesterol: 5mg
- Sodium: 20mg
- Carbohydrate: 10g
- Fiber: 2g
- Sugar: 7g
- Protein: 5g
- Vitamin C: 20%
- Calcium: 8%
- Iron: 1mg

Baked Cinnamon Apple Chips

Prep Time: 10 mins

Total Time: 2 hrs 10 mins

Servings: 4

Ingredients:

- 2 large apples, cored and thinly sliced

- 1 tablespoon honey or maple syrup
- 1 teaspoon ground cinnamon

Directions:

1. Preheat oven to 200°F (95°C). Line a baking sheet with parchment paper.
2. In a bowl, toss thinly sliced apples with honey or maple syrup and ground cinnamon until evenly coated.
3. Arrange the apple slices in a single layer on the prepared baking sheet.
4. Bake in the preheated oven for 2-3 hours, or until the apple slices are dried and crispy, flipping them halfway through.
5. Remove from the oven and let cool completely before serving.
6. Store any leftovers in an airtight container at room temperature for up to 3 days.

Nutrition Facts (per serving):

- Calories: 50
- Fat: 0g
- Saturated fat: 0g
- Cholesterol: 0mg
- Sodium: 0mg
- Carbohydrate: 14g
- Fiber: 2g
- Sugar: 11g
- Protein: 0g
- Vitamin C: 6%
- Calcium: 0%
- Iron: 0mg

Cottage Cheese and Pineapple Delight

Prep Time: 5 mins

Total Time: 5 mins

Servings: 1

Ingredients: 1/2 cup low-fat cottage cheese

- 1/2 cup diced pineapple
- 1 tablespoon chopped nuts (such as almonds or walnuts)
- 1 teaspoon honey or maple syrup (optional)

Directions:

1. In a bowl, combine low-fat cottage cheese and diced pineapple.
2. Sprinkle chopped nuts on top.
3. Drizzle with honey or maple syrup if desired.
4. Serve immediately as a refreshing snack or dessert.

Nutrition Facts (per serving):

- Calories: 150
- Fat: 5g
- Saturated fat: 1g
- Cholesterol: 10mg
- Sodium: 200mg
- Carbohydrate: 15g
- Fiber: 2g
- Sugar: 10g
- Protein: 12g
- Vitamin C: 80%
- Calcium: 15%
- Iron: 1mg

Dark Chocolate Covered Strawberries

Prep Time: 10 mins

Total Time: 30 mins

Servings: 4

Ingredients:

- 1 cup fresh strawberries, washed and dried
- 2 ounces dark chocolate, chopped
- 1 teaspoon coconut oil
- Optional toppings: chopped nuts, shredded coconut, sea salt

Directions:

1. Line a baking sheet with parchment paper.
2. In a microwave-safe bowl, combine chopped dark chocolate and coconut oil. Microwave in 30-second intervals, stirring in between, until chocolate is melted and smooth.
3. Dip each strawberry into the melted chocolate, coating about halfway.
4. Place the chocolate-covered strawberries on the prepared baking sheet.
5. Sprinkle optional toppings over the chocolate-covered strawberries if desired.
6. Refrigerate for 20 minutes, or until chocolate is set.
7. Serve immediately or store in the refrigerator for up to 2 days.

Nutrition Facts (per serving):

- Calories: 80
- Fat: 5g
- Saturated fat: 3g
- Cholesterol: 0mg

- Sodium: 0mg

- Carbohydrate: 9g

- Fiber: 2g

- Sugar: 6g

- Protein: 1g

- Vitamin C: 50%

- Calcium: 2%

- Iron: 1mg

Quinoa Protein Bites

Prep Time: 15 mins

Total Time: 30 mins

Servings: 12

Ingredients: 1 cup cooked quinoa

- 1/2 cup almond butter or peanut butter

- 1/4 cup honey or maple syrup

- 1/4 cup unsweetened shredded coconut

- 1/4 cup mini chocolate chips

- 1 teaspoon vanilla extract

- Pinch of salt

Directions:

1. In a large bowl, mix together cooked quinoa, almond butter or peanut butter, honey or maple syrup, unsweetened shredded coconut, mini chocolate chips, vanilla extract, and a pinch of salt until well combined.

2. Using your hands, roll the mixture into small balls, about 1 inch in diameter.

3. Place the quinoa protein bites on a baking sheet lined with parchment paper.

4. Refrigerate for at least 15 minutes to set.

5. Serve chilled as a nutritious snack or dessert.

Nutrition Facts (per serving - 2 bites):

- Calories: 160
- Fat: 9g
- Saturated fat: 3g
- Cholesterol: 0mg
- Sodium: 30mg
- Carbohydrate: 17g
- Fiber: 2g
- Sugar: 10g
- Protein: 4g
- Vitamin C: 0%
- Calcium: 2%
- Iron: 1mg

Veggie Stuffed Sweet Potato

Prep Time: 10 mins

Total Time: 1 hr 10 mins

Servings: 2

Ingredients:

- 2 medium sweet potatoes
- 1/2 cup black beans, drained and rinsed
- 1/2 cup corn kernels
- 1/4 cup diced bell pepper
- 1/4 cup diced red onion

- 1/4 cup chopped fresh cilantro
- 1 tablespoon lime juice
- 1/2 teaspoon ground cumin
- Salt and pepper to taste
- Optional toppings: avocado slices, Greek yogurt, salsa

Directions:

1. Preheat oven to 400°F (200°C). Line a baking sheet with parchment paper.
2. Scrub sweet potatoes and pierce several times with a fork. Place on the prepared baking sheet.
3. Bake sweet potatoes for 45-60 minutes, or until tender when pierced with a fork.
4. In a bowl, combine black beans, corn kernels, diced bell pepper, diced red onion, chopped fresh cilantro, lime juice, ground cumin, salt, and pepper. Mix well.
5. Once sweet potatoes are cooked, slice each one open lengthwise and fluff the flesh with a fork.
6. Stuff each sweet potato with the veggie mixture.
7. Serve immediately, topped with optional toppings if desired.

Nutrition Facts (per serving - 1 stuffed sweet potato):

- Calories: 250
- Fat: 1g
- Saturated fat: 0g
- Cholesterol: 0mg
- Sodium: 30mg
- Carbohydrate: 56g
- Fiber: 10g

- Sugar: 14g

- Protein: 8g

- Vitamin C: 100%

- Calcium: 6%

- Iron: 2mg

Greek Yogurt Parfait with Berries

Prep Time: 5 mins

Total Time: 5 mins

Servings: 1

Ingredients:

- 1/2 cup plain Greek yogurt

- 1/4 cup mixed berries (such as strawberries, blueberries, raspberries)

- 1 tablespoon honey or maple syrup

- 2 tablespoons granola

- Optional toppings: sliced almonds, shredded coconut, chia seeds

Directions:

1. In a glass or bowl, layer plain Greek yogurt, mixed berries, honey or maple syrup, and granola.

2. Repeat the layers until all ingredients are used up.

3. Top with optional toppings if desired.

4. Serve immediately as a satisfying snack or dessert.

Nutrition Facts (per serving):

- Calories: 250

- Fat: 5g

- Saturated fat: 0.5g

- Cholesterol: 5mg
- Sodium: 50mg
- Carbohydrate: 40g
- Fiber: 4g
- Sugar: 22g
- Protein: 15g
- Vitamin C: 20%
- Calcium: 15%
- Iron: 1mg

Baked Apple Chips

Prep Time: 10 mins

Total Time: 2 hrs 10 mins

Servings: 4

Ingredients:

- 2 apples (such as Fuji or Gala)
- 1 teaspoon ground cinnamon

Directions:

1. Preheat the oven to 200°F (95°C). Line a baking sheet with parchment paper.
2. Core and thinly slice the apples using a sharp knife or mandoline slicer.
3. Arrange the apple slices in a single layer on the prepared baking sheet.
4. Sprinkle ground cinnamon evenly over the apple slices.
5. Bake for 2 hours, flipping the slices halfway through, until the apples are dried and crisp.
6. Let the apple chips cool completely before serving.

7. Store any leftovers in an airtight container at room temperature for up to 3 days.

Nutrition Facts (per serving):

- Calories: 50
- Fat: 0g
- Saturated fat: 0g
- Cholesterol: 0mg
- Sodium: 0mg
- Carbohydrate: 14g
- Fiber: 2g
- Sugar: 11g
- Protein: 0g
- Vitamin C: 6%
- Calcium: 0%
- Iron: 0mg

Avocado Chocolate Mousse

Prep Time: 10 mins

Total Time: 10 mins

Servings: 2

Ingredients:

- 1 ripe avocado
- 2 tablespoons unsweetened cocoa powder
- 2 tablespoons honey or maple syrup
- 1/2 teaspoon vanilla extract
- Pinch of salt
- Optional toppings: sliced strawberries, shaved dark chocolate, whipped cream

Directions:

1. Scoop the flesh of the ripe avocado into a blender or food processor.
2. Add unsweetened cocoa powder, honey or maple syrup, vanilla extract, and a pinch of salt.
3. Blend until smooth and creamy, scraping down the sides as needed.
4. Divide the avocado chocolate mousse into serving glasses.
5. Chill in the refrigerator for at least 30 minutes before serving.
6. Top with optional toppings if desired.
7. Serve cold as a decadent dessert.

Nutrition Facts (per serving):

- Calories: 200
- Fat: 12g
- Saturated fat: 2g
- Cholesterol: 0mg
- Sodium: 5mg
- Carbohydrate: 26g
- Fiber: 7g
- Sugar: 16g
- Protein: 3g
- Vitamin C: 10%
- Calcium: 2%
- Iron: 1mg

Chia Seed Pudding

Prep Time: 5 mins

Total Time: 4 hrs 5 mins

Servings: 2

Ingredients:

- 1/4 cup chia seeds
- 1 cup unsweetened almond milk or coconut milk
- 1 tablespoon honey or maple syrup
- 1/2 teaspoon vanilla extract
- Optional toppings: fresh berries, sliced bananas, chopped nuts, shredded coconut

Directions:

1. In a bowl, combine chia seeds, unsweetened almond milk or coconut milk, honey or maple syrup, and vanilla extract.
2. Whisk together until well combined.
3. Cover the bowl and refrigerate for at least 4 hours or overnight, until the chia seeds have absorbed the liquid and the mixture has thickened.
4. Stir the chia seed pudding well before serving.
5. Divide the pudding into serving glasses.
6. Top with optional toppings if desired.
7. Serve chilled as a nutritious snack or dessert.

Nutrition Facts (per serving):

- Calories: 150
- Fat: 8g
- Saturated fat: 0.5g
- Cholesterol: 0mg

- Sodium: 80mg

- Carbohydrate: 16g

- Fiber: 10g

- Sugar: 4g

- Protein: 4g

- Vitamin C: 0%

- Calcium: 25%

- Iron: 2mg

Rice Cake with Almond Butter and Banana

Prep Time: 5 mins

Total Time: 5 mins

Servings: 1

Ingredients:

- 1 rice cake

- 1 tablespoon almond butter

- 1/2 banana, thinly sliced

- Optional toppings: drizzle of honey, sprinkle of cinnamon

Directions:

1. Spread almond butter evenly on top of the rice cake.

2. Arrange thinly sliced banana on top of the almond butter.

3. Drizzle with honey and sprinkle with cinnamon if desired.

4. Serve immediately as a quick and satisfying snack or dessert.

Nutrition Facts (per serving):

- Calories: 150

- Fat: 7g

- Saturated fat: 0.5g

- Cholesterol: 0mg

- Sodium: 60mg
- Carbohydrate: 19g
- Fiber: 3g
- Sugar: 7g
- Protein: 4g
- Vitamin C: 10%
- Calcium: 2%
- Iron: 1mg

Greek Yogurt Bark with Berries and Almonds

Prep Time: 10 mins

Total Time: 3 hrs 10 mins

Servings: 4

Ingredients:

- 1 cup plain Greek yogurt
- 1 tablespoon honey or maple syrup
- 1/4 cup mixed berries (such as strawberries, blueberries, raspberries)
- 2 tablespoons chopped almonds

Directions:

1. In a bowl, mix together plain Greek yogurt and honey or maple syrup until well combined.
2. Line a baking sheet with parchment paper.
3. Spread the Greek yogurt mixture evenly onto the prepared baking sheet.
4. Sprinkle mixed berries and chopped almonds over the Greek yogurt mixture, pressing them down lightly.
5. Freeze for at least 3 hours, or until firm.

6. Break the Greek yogurt bark into pieces.

7. Serve immediately as a refreshing snack or dessert.

Nutrition Facts (per serving):

- Calories: 80
- Fat: 4g
- Saturated fat: 0g
- Cholesterol: 0mg
- Sodium: 20mg
- Carbohydrate: 7g
- Fiber: 1g
- Sugar: 5g
- Protein: 6g
- Vitamin C: 10%
- Calcium: 8%
- Iron: 1mg

INCORPORATING EXERCISE FOR MAXIMUM RESULTS

Exercise Recommendations for Endomorph Women

Endomorph women often find themselves grappling with unique challenges when it comes to achieving their fitness goals. With a body type predisposed to retaining fat and building muscle, finding the right balance in exercise routines is crucial. However, it's essential to approach exercise not just as a means to an end but as a pathway to holistic well-being. In this chapter, we'll delve into exercise recommendations tailored specifically for endomorph women, focusing on fostering a positive mindset, building strength, and achieving sustainable results.

Understanding Your Body: Embracing Individual Differences

Before diving into exercise recommendations, it's vital for endomorph women to embrace their individual body types fully. Every woman's body is unique, and what works for one may not work for another. Rather than comparing yourself to others, focus on understanding your body's capabilities, strengths, and limitations. By embracing your uniqueness, you can tailor your exercise routine to suit your specific needs and preferences.

Finding Joy in Movement: Incorporating Variety

Exercise shouldn't feel like a chore; instead, it should be a source of joy and empowerment. Endomorph women can benefit from incorporating a variety of exercises into their routine to keep things interesting and engaging. From strength training and cardio to yoga and dance, explore different forms of movement to discover what resonates with you. By finding activities that you enjoy, you'll be more likely to stick to your exercise routine in the long run.

Strength Training: Building Lean Muscle Mass

One of the most effective forms of exercise for endomorph women is strength training. By building lean muscle mass, you can boost your metabolism and burn more calories throughout the day. Focus on compound exercises that target multiple muscle groups simultaneously, such as squats, deadlifts, lunges, and push-ups. Aim to incorporate strength training into your routine at least two to three times per week, gradually increasing the intensity as you progress.

Cardiovascular Exercise: Striking the Right Balance

While strength training is essential for endomorph women, cardiovascular exercise also plays a crucial role in achieving overall fitness and weight management. However, it's essential to strike the right balance and avoid overdoing it, as excessive cardio can lead to muscle loss and hinder progress. Instead, opt for moderate-intensity cardio activities such as brisk walking, cycling, swimming, or dancing. Aim for at least 150 minutes of moderate-intensity cardio per week, spread out over several days.

Mind-Body Practices: Cultivating Mindfulness and Relaxation

In addition to strength training and cardio, endomorph women can benefit from incorporating mind-body practices into their exercise routine. Practices such as yoga, Pilates, and tai chi not only improve flexibility, balance, and core strength but also promote relaxation and stress reduction. Prioritize incorporating these mindful movement practices into your routine to enhance your overall well-being and mental clarity.

Functional Fitness: Enhancing Daily Life

As an endomorph woman, it's essential to focus not just on aesthetics but also on functional fitness – the ability to perform everyday tasks with ease and efficiency. Incorporate functional exercises into your routine that mimic real-life movements, such as squats, lunges, and planks. By improving your functional strength and mobility, you'll enhance your quality of life and reduce the risk of injury.

Listen to Your Body: Prioritizing Rest and Recovery

Above all, listen to your body and prioritize rest and recovery. As an endomorph woman, your body may require more time to recover between workouts, so be sure to schedule rest days into your routine. Listen to your body's signals and adjust your exercise intensity and frequency accordingly. Remember that rest is just as important as exercise in achieving optimal health and fitness.

Strength Training vs. Cardio: Finding the Right Balance

Strength training, also known as resistance training or weightlifting, involves using external resistance – such as dumbbells, barbells, or resistance bands – to build muscle strength and endurance. Contrary to popular belief, strength training is not just for bodybuilders; it's essential for individuals of all fitness levels and goals.

One of the primary benefits of strength training is its ability to build lean muscle mass. As you engage in resistance exercises, you create microscopic tears in your muscle fibers, which then repair and grow stronger during the recovery process. Over time, this leads to increased muscle mass, improved muscle tone, and enhanced metabolic rate, ultimately resulting in greater calorie burn even at rest.

Strength training also offers numerous functional benefits, such as improved bone density, joint health, and balance, reducing the risk of injury and enhancing overall quality of life. Additionally, strength training can help alleviate symptoms of certain chronic conditions, such as arthritis, osteoporosis, and diabetes, making it a valuable component of a well-rounded fitness routine.

Exploring Cardiovascular Exercise: Boosting Heart Health

On the other hand, cardiovascular exercise, often referred to as cardio, focuses on elevating your heart rate and improving cardiovascular health. Common forms of cardio include running, cycling, swimming, and dancing, among others. Cardiovascular exercise primarily targets the cardiovascular system, including the heart, lungs, and circulatory system. Cardiovascular exercise offers a wide range of benefits, including improved heart health, increased endurance, and enhanced calorie burn. By elevating your heart rate and breathing rate, cardio helps strengthen your heart muscle, improve blood flow, and lower blood pressure, reducing the risk of heart disease and stroke. Additionally, regular cardio can boost mood, reduce stress, and improve mental clarity, making it beneficial for overall well-being.

Striking the Right Balance: Tailoring Your Routine

When it comes to strength training vs. cardio, there's no one-size-fits-all approach. The key is to tailor your exercise routine to align with your individual goals, preferences, and lifestyle. For some individuals, a balanced combination of strength training and cardio may be ideal, while others may prefer to focus more heavily on one or the other.

To strike the right balance, consider your fitness goals and prioritize exercises that align with them. If your goal is to build muscle and increase strength, prioritize strength training exercises such as weightlifting, bodyweight exercises, and resistance band workouts. Aim to incorporate strength training into your routine at least two to three times per week, targeting all major muscle groups for balanced development.

Alternatively, if your goal is to improve cardiovascular health, increase endurance, or burn calories, focus on incorporating cardio exercises into your routine. Choose activities that you enjoy and that you can sustain long term, whether it's running, cycling, swimming, or dancing. Aim for at least 150 minutes of moderate-intensity cardio per week, spread out over several days.

The Importance of Recovery and Rest

Regardless of whether you prioritize strength training, cardio, or a combination of both, it's crucial to prioritize recovery and rest. Muscles need time to repair and grow stronger after strength training sessions, while the cardiovascular system benefits from rest days to recover from intense cardio workouts. Incorporate rest days into your routine to prevent overtraining, reduce the risk of injury, and support overall recovery and well-being.

Integrating Physical Activity into Your Daily Routine

Finding time for exercise can often feel like an uphill battle. Between work commitments, family responsibilities, and other obligations, the idea of adding yet another item to your to-do list may seem overwhelming. However, incorporating physical activity into your daily routine doesn't have to be a daunting task. In fact, with a bit of creativity and intentionality, you can seamlessly integrate movement into your daily life, reaping the countless benefits that come with regular exercise.

Understanding the Importance of Physical Activity

Before delving into strategies for integrating physical activity into your daily routine, it's essential to understand why movement matters. Physical activity offers a myriad of benefits for both body and mind, ranging from improved cardiovascular health and weight management to enhanced mood and mental clarity. Regular exercise has been linked to a reduced risk of chronic diseases such as heart disease, diabetes, and certain types of cancer, making it a crucial component of a healthy lifestyle.

Furthermore, physical activity plays a vital role in maintaining muscle mass, bone density, and joint health as we age, helping to preserve mobility and independence. From boosting energy levels and promoting better sleep to reducing stress and anxiety, the benefits of regular exercise extend far beyond the physical realm, contributing to overall well-being and quality of life.

Identifying Opportunities for Movement

The first step in integrating physical activity into your daily routine is to identify opportunities for movement throughout the day. Instead of viewing exercise as a separate activity that requires dedicated time and effort, think of it as a natural part of your daily life. Look for ways to incorporate movement into activities you already do, such as walking or biking to work, taking the stairs instead of the elevator, or doing household chores like gardening or cleaning.

Additionally, consider incorporating short bursts of activity into your day, such as stretching or doing bodyweight exercises during work breaks, or taking a brisk walk during lunchtime. By breaking up prolonged periods of sitting with short bursts of movement, you can improve circulation, alleviate muscle tension, and boost energy levels throughout the day.

Making Movement a Priority

While it's easy to let exercise fall by the wayside amidst busy schedules and competing priorities, making movement a priority is essential for long-term health and well-being. Schedule regular exercise sessions into your calendar, treating them as non-negotiable appointments with yourself. Whether it's a morning yoga class, an evening jog, or a lunchtime walk, setting aside dedicated time for exercise helps ensure that it remains a consistent part of your routine.

Moreover, enlist the support of friends, family, or coworkers to hold you accountable and keep you motivated. Consider joining a group fitness class, participating in a sports team, or finding a workout buddy to keep you accountable and make exercise more enjoyable. By surrounding yourself with like-minded individuals who share your commitment to health and fitness, you can stay motivated and inspired on your journey toward a more active lifestyle.

Embracing Variety and Flexibility

Finally, remember that physical activity doesn't have to be limited to traditional forms of exercise like running or weightlifting. Embrace variety and flexibility in your approach to movement, exploring different activities and finding what works best for you. Whether it's dancing, swimming, cycling, or practicing martial arts, there are countless ways to move your body and stay active.

Furthermore, don't be afraid to adapt and modify your exercise routine based on your current circumstances and preferences. If time is limited, focus on shorter, more intense workouts that maximize efficiency and effectiveness. If you're recovering from an injury or dealing with physical limitations, explore low-impact exercises or alternative forms of movement that accommodate your needs.

OVERCOMING CHALLENGES AND STAYING MOTIVATED

Strategies for Overcoming Plateaus

A weight-loss plateau is when your weight stops changing. Being stuck at a weight-loss plateau eventually happens to everyone who tries to lose weight. Even so, most people are surprised when it happens to them because they're still eating carefully and exercising regularly. The frustrating reality is that even well-planned weight-loss efforts can stall. Plateaus are an inevitable part of any journey toward health and fitness. Whether you're striving to lose weight, build muscle, or improve your overall physical performance, hitting a plateau can be frustrating and disheartening. However, it's essential to remember that plateaus are not a sign of failure but rather an opportunity for growth and adaptation. By employing strategic approaches and staying committed to your goals, you can overcome plateaus and continue making progress on your wellness journey.

Understanding Plateaus: Why They Happen

Before diving into strategies for overcoming plateaus, it's crucial to understand why they occur in the first place. Plateaus typically occur when your body adapts to your current exercise and nutrition regimen, resulting in a temporary halt in progress. This adaptation can manifest in various ways, such as a stagnation in weight loss, a plateau in strength gains, or a lack of improvement in endurance or performance.

Plateaus can be caused by a variety of factors, including metabolic adaptation, insufficient recovery, inadequate nutrition, and lack of variety in your exercise routine. Additionally, psychological factors such as stress, boredom, or lack of motivation can also contribute to plateaus, making it essential to address both physical and mental aspects of your wellness journey.

Strategies for Overcoming Plateaus

1. **Modify Your Exercise Routine**: One of the most effective ways to overcome plateaus is to shake up your exercise routine. Incorporate new exercises, vary the intensity and duration of your workouts, and experiment with different training modalities such as high-intensity interval training (HIIT), circuit training, or plyometrics. By challenging your body in new ways, you can stimulate muscle growth, increase calorie burn, and break through plateaus.

2. **Increase Training Volume**: Another strategy for overcoming plateaus is to increase the volume of your training. This can involve performing more sets, repetitions, or training sessions per week, gradually increasing the workload to promote muscle hypertrophy and strength gains. However, it's essential to increase volume gradually and avoid overtraining, as this can lead to fatigue, injury, and burnout.

3. **Focus on Progressive Overload**: Progressive overload is the principle of gradually increasing the demands placed on the body during exercise to continually stimulate adaptation and progress. To overcome plateaus, focus on progressively increasing the intensity, volume, or complexity of your workouts over time. This can involve lifting heavier weights, performing more challenging

exercises, or increasing the duration or intensity of cardiovascular workouts.

4. **Prioritize Recovery**: Adequate recovery is essential for overcoming plateaus and maximizing performance. Ensure you're getting enough sleep, practicing stress management techniques, and incorporating rest days into your training schedule. Additionally, consider incorporating recovery modalities such as foam rolling, stretching, massage, or contrast baths to alleviate muscle soreness and enhance recovery between workouts.

5. **Fine-Tune Your Nutrition**: Nutrition plays a crucial role in overcoming plateaus and fueling performance. Evaluate your dietary habits and make adjustments as needed to support your goals. Focus on consuming a balanced diet rich in whole, nutrient-dense foods, and pay attention to factors such as portion sizes, macronutrient balance, and meal timing. Consider consulting with a registered dietitian or nutritionist for personalized guidance and support.

6. **Monitor Your Progress**: Keep track of your progress and performance to identify patterns and trends over time. Use tools such as workout logs, fitness apps, or wearable fitness trackers to monitor key metrics such as weight, body composition, strength, and endurance. By tracking your progress consistently, you can identify areas for improvement and make informed adjustments to your training and nutrition regimen.

7. **Stay Consistent and Patient**: Finally, remember that overcoming plateaus takes time, consistency, and patience. Stay committed to your goals, trust the process, and focus on making gradual improvements over time. Celebrate small victories along the way and stay resilient in the face of setbacks or challenges. By staying consistent and patient, you can overcome plateaus and continue making progress toward your health and fitness goals.

Dealing with Emotional Eating and Cravings

Emotional eating refers to the habit of using food to cope with or suppress negative emotions, rather than eating in response to physical hunger. It often involves consuming large quantities of high-calorie, highly palatable foods that provide temporary comfort or distraction from emotional distress. Emotional eating can stem from a variety of factors, including stress, anxiety, depression, boredom, loneliness, or unresolved emotional issues.

Identifying Triggers and Patterns

The first step in addressing emotional eating is to identify the triggers and patterns that contribute to it. Keep a food journal to track your eating habits and identify situations, emotions, or events that precede episodes of emotional eating. Pay attention to patterns and common triggers, such as stress at work, conflicts in relationships, or feelings of loneliness or boredom. By becoming more aware of your triggers, you can begin to develop strategies for managing them more effectively.

Coping Strategies for Emotional Eating

Once you've identified your triggers, it's essential to develop healthy coping strategies to manage them without turning to food. Experiment with alternative coping mechanisms such as exercise, meditation, deep breathing exercises, journaling, or engaging in hobbies or activities that bring you joy and fulfillment. Find healthy ways to soothe and comfort yourself that don't involve food, and practice self-compassion and self-care during times of emotional distress.

Mindful Eating Practices

Mindful eating involves paying attention to the sensory experience of eating and being fully present in the moment without judgment. Practice mindful eating by slowing down during meals, savoring each bite, and paying attention to the taste, texture, and aroma of your food. Tune into your body's hunger and fullness cues, and eat only when you're physically hungry, rather than in response to emotions or external cues. By practicing mindful eating, you can develop a more balanced and intuitive relationship with food and reduce the likelihood of emotional eating episodes.

Nutrition and Balanced Eating

Maintaining a balanced and nourishing diet is essential for managing cravings and preventing emotional eating. Focus on consuming a variety of whole, nutrient-dense foods such as fruits, vegetables, lean proteins, whole grains, and healthy fats. Include plenty of fiber-rich foods to promote satiety and stabilize blood sugar levels, which can help reduce cravings for sugary or high-calorie foods. Prioritize regular meals and snacks throughout the day to keep hunger and cravings in check, and avoid skipping meals or restricting food groups, which can lead to overeating and bingeing later on.

Seeking Support

If you find that emotional eating is significantly impacting your quality of life or ability to maintain a healthy diet, don't hesitate to seek support from a qualified healthcare professional or mental health therapist. Cognitive-behavioral therapy (CBT), mindfulness-based techniques, and other evidence-based approaches can be highly effective in helping individuals overcome emotional eating patterns and develop healthier coping mechanisms. Additionally, joining a support group or seeking support from friends, family members, or peers who understand your struggles can provide invaluable encouragement and accountability on your journey toward better health.

Cultivating a Positive Mindset for Long-Term Success

Achieving and maintaining long-term success in any endeavor, including health and wellness, requires more than just following a set of rules or guidelines. It requires a positive mindset—a mental outlook that empowers you to overcome challenges, stay motivated, and persevere in the face of setbacks. In this chapter, we'll explore the importance of cultivating a positive mindset for long-term success on your journey toward better health and wellness.

The Power of Positive Thinking

Positive thinking is more than just wishful thinking or blind optimism. It's a mindset that focuses on possibilities, solutions, and opportunities rather than dwelling on problems or limitations. Research has shown that cultivating a positive mindset can have numerous benefits for physical and mental health, including reduced stress, improved immune function, enhanced resilience, and greater overall well-being.

Challenging Negative Beliefs and Self-Talk

One of the first steps in cultivating a positive mindset is to become aware of and challenge negative beliefs and self-talk that may be holding you back. Pay attention to your inner dialogue and notice when you're engaging in negative or self-defeating thoughts. Replace these negative thoughts with more positive and empowering affirmations. For example, instead of saying, "I'll never be able to lose weight," try saying, "I am capable of making healthy choices and reaching my goals."

Practicing Gratitude and Mindfulness

Gratitude and mindfulness are powerful practices that can help shift your mindset from one of scarcity to one of abundance and appreciation. Take time each day to reflect on the things you're grateful for, whether it's your health, relationships, accomplishments, or simple pleasures like a beautiful sunset or a delicious meal. Practicing mindfulness—being fully present in the moment without judgment—can also help cultivate a positive mindset by helping you focus on the here and now rather than worrying about the future or dwelling on the past.

Setting Realistic Goals and Celebrating Progress

Setting realistic, achievable goals is essential for maintaining motivation and momentum on your journey toward better health. Break your larger goals down into smaller, manageable steps, and celebrate your progress along the way. Recognize and celebrate even the smallest victories, whether it's making healthier food choices, sticking to your exercise routine, or overcoming a particular challenge. Celebrating your progress reinforces positive behaviors and builds confidence, making it easier to stay motivated and committed to your goals in the long term.

Surrounding Yourself with Positive Influences

The people you surround yourself with can have a significant impact on your mindset and outlook on life. Surround yourself with positive, supportive individuals who uplift and encourage you on your journey toward better health. Seek out mentors, friends, or family members who share your goals and values and who can provide guidance, inspiration, and accountability along the way. Limit your exposure to negative influences, whether it's toxic relationships, negative media, or environments that undermine your efforts to cultivate a positive mindset.

LONG-TERM MAINTENANCE AND LIFESTYLE CHANGES

Transitioning from a Diet to a Sustainable Lifestyle

Diets often come with strict rules, restrictions, and guidelines that can be difficult to maintain over the long term. They often promote rapid weight loss through calorie restriction or elimination of certain food groups, leading to feelings of deprivation, frustration, and ultimately, failure. Moreover, diets tend to focus solely on the physical aspects of health, neglecting the importance of mental, emotional, and social well-being.

Embracing a Sustainable Lifestyle

Unlike diets, which are typically short-term and focused on achieving a specific outcome, a sustainable lifestyle encompasses long-term, holistic changes that promote overall health and well-being. It involves making gradual, sustainable changes to eating habits, physical activity, stress management, and self-care practices. Rather than viewing health as a destination to be reached, it's about embracing health as a journey—an ongoing process of growth, learning, and self-discovery.

Making Gradual Changes

Transitioning from a diet to a sustainable lifestyle begins with making gradual, sustainable changes to your eating habits and daily routines. Instead of following strict rules or eliminating entire food groups, focus on incorporating more whole, nutrient-dense foods into your diet, such as fruits, vegetables, lean proteins, and whole grains. Experiment with new recipes, flavors, and cooking techniques to keep meals interesting and satisfying.

Listening to Your Body

One of the key principles of transitioning to a sustainable lifestyle is learning to listen to your body's hunger and fullness cues. Rather than relying on external rules or guidelines to dictate when and what to eat, tune in to your body's signals and eat mindfully. Pay attention to how different foods make you feel, both physically and emotionally, and make choices that nourish and energize you.

Finding Joy in Movement

Physical activity is an essential component of a sustainable lifestyle, but it doesn't have to feel like punishment or obligation. Instead of forcing yourself to adhere to a rigid exercise routine, find activities that you enjoy and that fit seamlessly into your daily life. Whether it's dancing, hiking, swimming, or practicing yoga, choose activities that bring you joy and make you feel good, rather than focusing solely on burning calories or achieving a certain physique.

Cultivating Self-Compassion

Transitioning to a sustainable lifestyle requires patience, persistence, and self-compassion. Understand that setbacks and challenges are a natural part of the process and that it's okay to stumble along the way. Rather than being hard on yourself for perceived failures or slip-ups, practice self-compassion and treat yourself with kindness and understanding. Remember that every step you take towards a healthier lifestyle, no matter how small, is progress in the right direction.

Strategies for Maintaining Weight Loss

Achieving weight loss is often seen as a significant milestone in one's health journey, but the real challenge lies in maintaining that weight loss over the long term. In this chapter, we'll explore various strategies for maintaining weight loss and building a sustainable lifestyle that supports your health and well-being.

Understanding the Challenges

Maintaining weight loss can be challenging for many reasons. After reaching their weight loss goals, some individuals may revert to old habits, leading to weight regain. Additionally, the body's metabolism may adapt to the lower calorie intake, making it harder to continue losing weight or maintain weight loss. Moreover, emotional and environmental factors, such as stress, social gatherings, and food availability, can also influence eating behaviors and contribute to weight regain.

Focus on Sustainable Habits

Rather than relying on restrictive diets or short-term solutions, focus on building sustainable habits that support your long-term health and well-being. This includes adopting a balanced and varied diet rich in whole, nutrient-dense foods, such as fruits, vegetables, lean proteins, and whole grains. Incorporate regular physical activity into your daily routine and find activities that you enjoy and can maintain over the long term.

Monitor Your Progress

Monitoring your progress is essential for maintaining weight loss and staying accountable to your goals. Keep track of your food intake, physical activity, and weight on a regular basis. This can help you identify patterns, recognize areas for improvement, and make necessary adjustments to your lifestyle. Additionally, monitoring your progress can provide motivation and encouragement as you see the positive changes taking place.

Stay Consistent

Consistency is key when it comes to maintaining weight loss. Stick to your healthy eating and exercise habits even when life gets busy or challenging. Plan ahead and prioritize your health by making time for meal prep, scheduling regular workouts, and finding ways to stay active throughout the day. Remember that small, consistent actions add up to significant results over time.

Manage Stress and Emotions

Stress and emotions can have a significant impact on eating behaviors and weight management. Learn healthy coping mechanisms for managing stress, such as mindfulness, deep breathing, or engaging in hobbies and activities that bring you joy. Practice self-care and prioritize your mental and emotional well-being as part of your overall health routine.

Build a Support Network

Having a support network can make a significant difference in maintaining weight loss. Surround yourself with friends, family, or support groups who share similar health goals and can provide encouragement, accountability, and motivation along the way. Share your successes, challenges, and experiences with others, and celebrate each other's progress together.

Be Kind to Yourself

Lastly, remember to be kind to yourself throughout your weight maintenance journey. Recognize that setbacks and challenges are a natural part of the process, and treat yourself with compassion and understanding. Avoid self-criticism or negative self-talk, and instead, focus on the progress you've made and the positive changes you've implemented in your life.

Building Healthy Habits for Life

Habits are the foundation of our daily lives. They are the routines and behaviors that we perform automatically, often without conscious thought. Whether it's brushing your teeth in the morning, going for a daily walk, or reaching for a healthy snack instead of junk food, habits play a significant role in shaping our health and lifestyle choices.

Start Small and Be Consistent

When it comes to building healthy habits, starting small is key. Instead of trying to overhaul your entire lifestyle overnight, focus on making small, manageable changes that you can sustain over time. Whether it's adding an extra serving of vegetables to your meals, taking the stairs instead of the elevator, or committing to a daily meditation practice, choose one or two habits to focus on initially and gradually build from there.

Consistency is also essential when it comes to building healthy habits. Make a commitment to practice your chosen habit every day, even if it's just for a few minutes. Over time, these small actions will add up, and you'll start to see significant improvements in your health and well-being.

Set Clear Goals

Setting clear, achievable goals is another crucial aspect of building healthy habits for life. Identify what you want to accomplish and why it's important to you. Whether your goal is to lose weight, improve your fitness level, or reduce stress, having a clear sense of purpose will help keep you motivated and focused on your journey.

Break down your larger goals into smaller, actionable steps, and track your progress along the way. Celebrate your successes and be gentle with yourself if you encounter setbacks. Remember that building healthy habits is a journey, not a destination, and it's okay to adjust your goals and strategies as needed.

Create a Supportive Environment

Building healthy habits is much easier when you have a supportive environment that encourages and reinforces your efforts. Surround yourself with people who share similar health goals and values, whether it's friends, family members, or online communities. Seek out resources and tools that support your journey, such as healthy recipes, workout programs, or meditation apps.

Additionally, make changes to your physical environment to make healthy choices easier and more convenient. Keep nutritious foods stocked in your kitchen, set up a designated workout space at home, and remove any temptations or obstacles that may derail your progress.

Practice Mindfulness and Self-Compassion

Mindfulness and self-compassion are essential tools for building healthy habits for life. Cultivate awareness of your thoughts, feelings, and behaviors, and practice being present in the moment. Notice any patterns or triggers that may lead to unhealthy habits, and explore healthier alternatives.

Be kind and compassionate with yourself throughout your journey. Accept that setbacks and challenges are a natural part of the process, and treat yourself with the same kindness and understanding that you would offer to a friend. Remember that building healthy habits is not about perfection but about progress and self-improvement.

CONCLUSION

In the pursuit of optimal health and wellness, embarking on the Metabolism Reset Diet for Endomorph Women represents a significant step towards achieving your goals. Throughout this comprehensive guide, we've explored a myriad of topics, ranging from understanding endomorph body types to strategies for maintaining weight loss. Each chapter has been meticulously crafted to provide you with the knowledge, tools, and motivation necessary to embark on a transformative journey towards a healthier, happier you.

As endomorph women, we understand the unique challenges and frustrations that come with striving to achieve our health and fitness goals. From grappling with stubborn body fat to navigating emotional eating and cravings, the road to success is often littered with obstacles. However, armed with the insights and strategies outlined in this guide, you possess the power to overcome these challenges and emerge victorious in your pursuit of a balanced, vibrant lifestyle.

One of the key takeaways from this journey is the importance of adopting a holistic approach to health and wellness. By addressing not only dietary habits and exercise routines but also mindset, emotional well-being, and lifestyle factors, you can create a sustainable foundation for long-term success. It's about more than just numbers on a scale or inches lost; it's about cultivating a positive relationship with yourself, nourishing your body, and embracing the journey of self-discovery and growth.

Throughout this guide, we've emphasized the significance of self-compassion and resilience in the face of setbacks. We understand that progress is not always linear and that there may be bumps along the road.

However, it's in these moments of challenge and adversity that we have the opportunity to learn, grow, and ultimately emerge stronger than ever before. Remember, it's not about perfection; it's about progress. Celebrate your victories, no matter how small, and use your setbacks as stepping stones towards greater success.

As you embark on this transformative journey, keep in mind the words of Henry Ford: "Whether you think you can or you think you can't, you're right." Believe in yourself, trust in your abilities, and have faith in the power of your own resilience. You are capable of achieving anything you set your mind to, and with dedication, determination, and a positive mindset, there's no limit to what you can accomplish.

So, as you continue on your path towards health and wellness, remember to be gentle with yourself, celebrate your progress, and embrace the journey with open arms. You have everything you need to succeed within you; all that's left is to take that first step and embark on the adventure of a lifetime. Here's to your health, happiness, and endless potential. The world is yours for the taking—go out there and make it yours.

"Believe you can, and you're halfway there." - Theodore Roosevelt